MW01703093

Dual Diagnosis Dialogue

Dual Diagnosis Dialogue

First Edition

Publisher: Independent Publisher Services, Chicago, IL 60611

Author: Scott L.Gourson LPC, MS, LADC, CCDP, CAC

Assistant Editor: Seth S. Gourson

Composition and Cover Design: William W. Semrau
www.bwsgraphics.com

ISBN: 978-1-4507-6060-7

ISBN: 978-1-4507-5678-5 (paperback)

E-mail: sgourson@comcast.net

Web: www.scottgourson.com

Independent Publisher Services
875 North Michigan Ave.
Chicago, IL 60611

Dual Diagnosis Dialogue

A Handbook and Overview
For the Entry Level Substance Use Counselor

By Scott L. Gourson LPC, MS, LADC, CCDP, CAC

Assistant Editor: Seth S. Gourson

Dedication

This Book is dedicated to the still sick and suffering individuals with a co-occurring disorder who have not yet been fortunate to find recovery.

Also, in loving memory of Dad . . .
and in loving honor of Mom.

Acknowledgement

Special thanks to my son, Seth, for his conscientious and expeditious efforts assisting in fine editorial detail.

Contents

Contents

Contents

Contents

Contents

Comment for the Reader

About This Book

This book is written from various perspectives – professional, researcher, and personal. It is the culmination of my pursuits on these levels. My purpose is to present an easy-to-read guide for the beginner counselor, and those who want a concise and basic overview and reference handbook that highlights fundamental areas of dual diagnosis counseling. I've tried to write it as though you were sitting in the room with me and I have tried to keep it simple, yet scholarly. My experience is that folks come into substance abuse counseling with various levels of education and experience – particularly recovering individuals – and I largely have you in mind. Your instincts are good and your heart is in the right place or you wouldn't have gotten this far! It is my hope that you can benefit from a review of need-to-know professional topics to enhance your intuitive counseling skills. Over 60% of our substance use clients have another mental health diagnosis; they always did, but we know more now and this is how we view things today (Inaba & Cohen, 2004). Integrated treatment, simultaneously addressing both the substance usage and the other mental health diagnoses, is becoming the standard in the field. Integrated treatment has its own approach or paradigm, a blend of both mental health and substance use counseling. The book is a combination of background and history, counseling theory and diagnostic data, physiology, and a view of today's paths to recovery. I hope it is useful and fun! God bless.

UNIT 1/Addiction Theory

Introduction

This unit discusses various perspectives regarding addiction. What is important to keep in mind is that theories may seem contradictory and opposing. However, there really is room for all schools of thought as there are certainly cases where all are applicable. I have included histories of drug usage, treatment, and recovery as well as the story of Alcoholics Anonymous. Hopefully, they help to demonstrate how today's perspectives in the field were developed. Harm reduction theory is presented here because it was important to introduce this idea early in the book, as it has relevance in many areas. It is a very provocative and controversial issue, and would seemingly go against everything we know about recovery. See what you think.

CHAPTER 1

Addiction Theory

> *Comment for the Reader:* Let me say from the start that this book uses various terms interchangeably: 1) alcoholism and addiction. As far as I'm concerned, alcoholism is addiction. The distinction has been a historical one. 2) Alcoholic and addict. Again, same idea. 3) The terms *dual diagnosis, co-morbid condition*, and *co-occurring disorders* all refer to a substance abuse issue combined with another mental health condition.

While broad research has been studied, there is no consensus on the origins of addiction/alcoholism. However, the research seems to concentrate in three areas: biological, psychological, and socio-cultural/environmental. Biological theories include the disease model, genetic predisposition, and the effects of other biological factors. The disease model has been widely accepted by the medical profession and forms the basis of many treatment programs, including Alcoholics Anonymous (Alcoholics Anonymous, 1939; Jellinek, 1960). This approach advocates complete abstinence and indicates that dependency is characterized by out-of-control usage, which is progressive and declining in course (APA, 2004). A genetic theory is supported by research that often alcoholism runs higher in families than in the general population (Lawson, et al., 1983). Other research that supports alcoholism is due to certain biological factors found in alcoholics but not in non-alcoholics; i.e., higher levels of acetaldehyde (an organic compound) and lower levels of serotonin (Ait-Douad, 2009). Examples of psychological theories include personality theories; i.e., the "addictive" personality which is suggested by higher levels of impulsiveness, aggression, emotionality, agitation, and frustration (Eysenk, 1991). Psychodynamic theory might suggest that alcoholism is not a disease, but rather psychological symptoms that become a physical addiction (Corey, 2009). Behavior and learning theories might suggest that addiction is not a disease but learned behavior (Corey, 2009). Socio-cultural theories suggest that because alcohol consumption is considered socially acceptable, social attitudes may be related to alcoholism. Drug abusers are often susceptible to peer pressure (Johnson, 2007; Quintero, 2006). The availability of alcohol and other drugs is another factor.

> *Comment for the Reader:* It is important to know today that the medical model, supported by 12-Step programs is not the ONLY way to look at things. There was a real tendency to pigeonhole people into a one size fits all theory, and therefore subsequent treatment. People have problems with drugs for many reasons, and there are many ways to approach treatment and recovery. There is no wrong way to recover.

CHAPTER 2

The Addictive Personality: Fact or Fiction?

The addictive personality. There isn't one. At least we cannot prove it empirically, anyway, with quantitative methodology research. Most of the research on the theory of an addictive personality was from 1960-1985. The problem is, although we may feel that a certain type of person becomes addicted, there are too many personality factors with too many qualitative and quantitative variables to say when a person has this trait and that trait, with this factor and that factor, they will become addicted. That is because it may not be true all the time; or there are other times when it is due to different factors; or this person has all these factors but not this one, but has that one over here. So I think you get the idea: there is insufficient consistency to develop a scientific profile.

However, in the process we have learned a lot and a lot of useful information has emerged. For example, we know that neuroticism is associated with addiction (Eysenk, 1994). We know that addiction is associated with reward dependence (something like a reliance on immediate gratification)(Sher, Bartolow, & Wood, 2000). We know that alcohol usage is correlated with excitement seeking (Mustanski et al., 2003). And we have learned a myriad of other factors relevant to addiction as well.

The addictive personality is a favorite topic of mine and so I include it here. It is safe to say that addicts/alcoholics have a certain "X" factor. This is not a new or original concept. Addicts/alcoholics do seem to have something going on that makes them have a propensity or an inclination toward addiction and it is worth taking a further look at here.

The field of addiction has been considered to be "an ideological battlefield" (I love that phrase) when it comes to identifying the addictive personality (Sutker & Allain, 1988, p. 174). Little consensus can be found to explain the etiology (cause) and expression of addiction and there remain, after some 50 years of modern research, considerable questions concerning concepts of personality and addictive behaviors. The idea that genetic or constitutional factors are a part of the addiction process is not new. Sutker & Allain cite Crothers and Sudduth dating back to the late 1800s.

After a cursory review of later literature dating from the 1940s, three general conflicting perspectives are cast into a basic framework, which is the source of controversy over the validity of the addictive personality (Vaillant, 1995):

1) Addiction is precipitated by psychopathology that is characterized by a set of specific personality characteristics. In other words, addiction is caused by personality or perhaps temperament.

2) Addiction is not necessarily caused by or correlated to psychopathology, character defects, or specific traits.

3) Aberrant personality traits are the result of, not the cause of, alcoholism/addiction.

There are many arguments arising from researching the addictive personality. Initially, what population is being researched? I am most interested in the personality that precedes alcohol/drug use. However, most research has examined those who are already alcoholic/addicted, or in treatment, or maintaining sobriety. This research then raises the question – did personality traits found in this population precede chemical dependence or are a result of it ? Each group is a separate population with potentially different personality characteristics.

Or, are there prevalent or enduring qualities which are stable that precipitate and are supported into active addiction/alcoholism (Kinney & Leaton, 1987)?

The question becomes – are there personality traits or combinations thereof that differ for abusers and non-abusers? What are the differences in personality development and expression that change over the life span? Lastly, what are internal factors and how do they influence the addictive personality theories?

First, let's look at common and similar findings from research on the addictive personality through a framework of major theories. We will then go on to discuss the relevancy and applications in substance abuse counseling.

Addictive Personality Traits

Pervin, Cervone, & Oliver (2005) discuss Hans Eysenck. Eysenck discusses 3 basic dimensions of personality: Introversion vs. extraversion, stability vs. instability (neuroticism), and social vs. anti-social (psychoticism). Eysenck (1991) states that neuroticism is largely inheritable; also that anxiety and depression are largely influenced by environmental factors.

Characteristic of Eysenck's views, is his focus on a small number of personality types. For him, types are not categories that people fit in. Instead, they are dimensions along which people differ. One need not be either an introvert or an extravert; instead, one can fall anywhere along a continuum ranging from extreme introversion on one end to extreme extraversion at the other. Most people would fall somewhere in the middle.

Eysenck was influenced by the concept of temperament, which lies underneath personality. Temperament provides a broader perspective than personality (Horton & Oakland, 1997). The four purported temperaments are: sanguine (cheerful, confident), melancholic (gloomy), choleric (angry), and phlegmatic (apathetic). To support these ideas, Eysenck gathered data based on ratings of subjects. In the end, information from thousands of subjects was examined and the results convinced him of the existence and usefulness of the three above dimensions. Eysenck believed that not only are the temperaments shown in relation to the dimension types, but also a series of trait-like adjectives further define the characteristics with each type (Eysenck & Rachman, 1975). In other words, Eysenk draws on the relationship between temperment (which refers to innate qualities) and personality (which refers to types, traits, and individual differences). Many researchers use Eysenck's theories.

Tarter (1988) talks in terms of 'emotionality.' This is a propensity toward becoming easily and intensely distressed. These correlate to Eysenck's scales of stability and introversion. Alcoholics often score higher than non-alcoholics on the neuroticism dimension, but not on the introversion-extroversion scale (alcoholics tend to be more introverted). Tarter also draws a relationship between neuroticism and genetic causes.

In terms of sociability, Tarter (1988) reports that alcoholics are "bold, uninhibited, self-confident, social, people who mix well with others." This writer assumes he is talking about the active alcoholic. In most cases, the writer believes, the antedated alcoholic may not look that way.

Sher & Trull (1994) review empirical findings for Eysenck's scales. They refer to them as neuroticism/emotionality, impulsivity/disinhibition, and extraversion/sociability. Then they look at theoretical models for both dependence and anti-social personality. While etiology and/or correlation are not drawn, it is concluded, in agreement with Eysenk, that personality variables are important components.

Perhaps this is as close as we get to define the addictive personality. That is, to just be able to say that personality components are important when looking at dependence. Vaillant (1995) provides the impression that there are too many characteristics with too many factors with too many variables to determine etiology of dependence.

Sher & Trull (1994) come up with a working definition of personality as "internal, unique, enduring, active, causal, and integrating (p. 93)." The problem was a number of individual-differences variables that have been associated with alcoholism do not meet the criteria as set forth by the personality theories. For example, traits shown to be associated with anti-sociability (like a history of behavior problems) are a high predictor of an alcohol problem, but are not necessarily causal.

Sher, Bartholow, & Wood (2000) use Cloninger's Big Three Personality Systems,which is a spin-off of Eysenck. Cloninger's three systems (of personality traits) are harm avoidance, reward dependence, and novelty-seeking. Harm avoidance is described as cautious, apprehensible, fatiguable, inhibited, and sensitive to punishment. Reward dependence is described as ambitious, sympathetic, warm, industrious, sentimental, persistent, and moody. Novelty seeking is described as impulsive, excitable, exploratory, quick-tempered, fickle, extravagant, and disinhibited.

Mustanski et al., (2003) correlate excitement-seeking with alcohol consumption. Excitement seeking is like Cloninger's novelty-seeking, which is like Eysenck's extraversion. Slutske et al., (2002) correlate alcohol dependence with conduct disorder. Conduct disorder would be high on Eysenck's psychoticism dimension.

A study by McGue, Slutske, & Iacono (1999) demonstrates some of the confounding factors involved with drawing conclusions from a study. The study included 638 individuals who were alcoholic and/or had a drug use disorder. Two questions of reliability and validity arise at this juncture: 1) Is the antedated drinker different than the current drinker? 2) Are there differences between a drinker, drug abuser, and co-addicted individual? Data was analyzed from 3 factors: gender, alcoholism, drug use disorder. What about age? The study is an example of issues that researchers run into when studying addiction/alcoholism.

The significant trait associated with alcoholism is negative emotionality (or high on Eysenck's neuroticism dimension). The significant trait associated with drug use disorder is constraint. This also falls on the neuroticism continuum. No significant findings were drawn from gender. Also, findings suggest that drug use disorder individuals had higher levels of behavioral disinhibition than those who drank alcohol. This is not necessarily what this writer would expect. However, it may depend upon what drug was being used.

Hendriks (1990) did a study involving 152 participants in a detoxification center. At least 80% also carried a psychiatric disorder. The three most diagnosed disorders were anti-social personality, depressive disorder, and anxiety-related disorder. Often, they were diagnosed in combination of each other. Almost half of those diagnosed with anti-social disorder were also diagnosed with a depressive or anxiety disorder. Those with longer drug use histories had anti-social personalities. Does this imply continued drug use causes/enhances/simply correlates with anti-social personality?

Along these lines, Nathan (1988) distinguishes between anti-social behavior and anti-social personality. His studies reveal a correlation between anti-social behaviors in childhood and adolescence, and alcoholism as an adult. However, because there are such high rates of anti-social behavior, it cannot be considered causal or even a predictor of alcoholism. No personality factors or behaviors consistently differentiate between abusers and non-abusers.

Kagan (2001) devised a study using the MacAndrew Alcoholism Scale collecting mean scores comparing alcoholics to compulsive gamblers, smokers, chronic joggers, and control subjects on six factors: social maladjustment, cognitive impairment, risk taking, extroversion, moral indignation, and interpersonal competence. A compulsiveness scale was also used: indecision and double-checking, order and regularity, detail and perfectionism. Alcoholics scored higher in all areas as the most pathological group; the six personality factors above figure in to a description of an addictive personality.

Kerr (1996) makes some interesting observations and raises some interesting questions. His review of the literature summarizes personality features of alcoholics/addicts. They include: "low self-esteem; marked sensitivity to expressions of approval or disapproval; high anxiety; low frustration tolerance; hedonism; helplessness; ineptitude; lack of friends, gregariousness; being loners; guilt; futility; depressiveness; dependence; demanding attention; immaturity; psychopathy; impulsiveness, shyness, aggression; non-aggression; soft-spokenness, verbally adept; pleasant; likeable; and sociable, with an interest to the arts, particularly music; (p. S10)." Kerr (1996) states that the list could continue and it could describe the average person and anyone with psychiatric difficulties. This writer does not agree that it describes the average person. This list is more skewed than that toward higher dimensions of these qualities. Nonetheless, the list is broad and rather general.

Kerr (1996) cites Rozin and Stoess (1993) and raises the question: "[if there is not an addictive personality per se, then] Is addiction based on tendency at all? (p. S10)?" This is a fascinating question. However, their study indicated there is little basis for this assumption. But, if personality does not cause addiction, then what does?

Kerr purports that causative factors probably prominently include emotional problems from genetic or childhood experiences. If it does, in fact, the next question is whether personality changes over time (Kerr, 1996).

Kerr (1996) states that the argument for the addictive personality is based on out-dated, naïve perspectives of the personality; that it does not include more recent ideas such as locus of control (the extent to which people believe they can control things that affect their lives), risk-taking, and sensation-seeking. He also believes there are other environmental and learning factors which are present.

Sutker and Allain (1988) report psychoanalytic explanations for addiction, such as "regression, developmental lags, the pleasure principle, and painful mental states (p. 175)." In other words, they cite Khantzian (1982, 1985), who argues addicts use drugs to quiet, contain, or obviate the rage and aggression that is prevalent in the personality.

EYSENCK'S THEORIES ON ADDICTION

Eysenck (1997) takes a very matter-of-fact approach to the question of an addictive personality. He purports that there is evidence that all aspects of personality are determined genetically. He states DNA does not cause our behavior, but that there are links called biological intermediaries between our DNA and our behavior. Furthermore, this relationship can predict "distal consequences (physiological effects) (p. 80)." He believes the psychoticism dimension is most closely correlated with addictive behavior and to a smaller extent, neuroticism and lower levels of extraversion.

Based on this information, Gossop & Eysenck (1980) constructed a 32-item Addiction Scale. Addicts have scores almost twice the mean of the control individuals.

1) Do you stop to think things over before doing anything?
2) Does your mood often go up and down?
3) Do you ever feel 'just miserable' for no reason?
4) Were you ever greedy by helping yourself to more than your share of anything?
5) Do you lock up your house carefully at night?
6) If you say you will do something, do you always keep your promise no matter how inconvenient it may be?

7) Can you usually let yourself go and enjoy yourself at a lively party?

8) Do you enjoy meeting new people?

9) Do you believe insurance schemes are a good idea?

10) Would you take drugs, which have strange and dangerous effects?

11) Do you often feel 'fed up'?

12) Have you ever taken anything (even a pin or button) that belonged to someone else?

13) Are you often troubled by feelings of guilt?

14) Do you have enemies that want to harm you?

15) Would you call yourself a nervous person?

16) Do you have many friends?

17) Are you a worrier?

18) Would you call yourself tense or 'high-strung'?

19) Do you like mixing with people?

20) Do you suffer from sleeplessness?

21) Have you often felt listless and tired for no reason?

22) Is (or was) your mother a good woman?

23) Do you often feel life is very dull?

24) Have you ever taken advantage of someone?

25) Are there several people trying to avoid you?

26) Have you ever wished that you were dead?

27) Would you dodge paying taxes if you were sure you could never be found out?

28) When you catch a train do you often arrive at the last minute?

29) Do you suffer from 'nerves'?

30) Do your friendships break up easily without it being your fault?

31) Do you often feel lonely?

32) Have you ever been late for an appointment or work?

Almost half are drawn from the Neuroticism scale. Nine out of the 32 are taken from the psychoticism scale. Questions 1, 5, 9, 27, and 28 are seen as a willingness to defy convention. Six questions were taken from a Lie Scale and four were taken from an Extraversion Scale.

Addicts scored higher than control individuals and females scored slightly higher than males. Addicts clearly regard themselves as nervous, sensitive, and moody. The results indicate many addicts feel that drugs help them cope with their problems. And most of these problems have a high neurotic component. Implications are that addicts use drugs to counteract a lack of confidence and social anxiety.

These studies were performed on people in treatment. Gossop & Eysenck (1997) wonder if neurotic symptoms of clients were "rewarded." Did clients receive more praise and attention from staff and peers for bringing up these items? Is it possible that clients leave with more symptoms than they came in with? Such questions point out other difficulties in describing the addictive personality.

Eysenck (1997) goes on to say that two dimensions are related to etiology.

The first relates to psychoticism with qualities like impulsivity, inattention, and character disorders. The other is neuroticism or negative emotion factors with a propensity toward negative moral states and psychological distress.

Eysenck (1997) believes there are biological antecedents of addiction. Drugs characterized with abuse and dependence are all able to "increase neurotransmission in the mesolimbic dopamine system (p. 83)." Various addictive drugs, such as cocaine, amphetamines, alcohol, morphine, and nicotine raise dopamine levels (which make people feel good).

Furthermore, Eysenck (1997) cites Fowler (1996) with linking addiction and dopamine activity. Smokers show a decrease in monoamine oxidase (MAO), which breaks down dopamine. MAO inhibitors are associated with high dopamine activity. Low MAO levels are associated with psychopathology. There is a prevalence of smoking among psychiatric disorders. Thus dopamine is associated with psychoticism scoring. Eysenck (1997) calls this the "fundamental link between personality and biology (p. 84)."

Eysenck (1997) suggest this data is the general basis for addiction. To take it a step further, the mesolimbic dopamine system (dopamine pathways in the brain) is associated with the principle of reward and reinforcement. Drugs of abuse produce an increase in dopamine. It's simple. Addiction occurs because the drugs produce reinforcing factors in the brain (Eysenck, 1997). Eysenck concludes that the dopamine system plays a general role in addiction, reward, and motivation.

One problem with this theory is that various animal studies associated with increased dopamine demonstrate that it produces stress and aversive stimuli as well as reward. Thus it also contains a punishing factor as well (Eysenck, 1997).

VAILLANT'S THOUGHTS ON ALCOHOLISM

George Vaillant is a Professor of Psychiatry at Harvard Medical School. His first book, *The Natural History of Alcoholism*, discusses crucial questions of whether alcoholism is a symptom or a disease, whether it is progressive, whether alcoholics differ from others before the onset of their alcoholism, and whether alcoholics can drink safely (without negative consequences).

Vaillant (1995) states that there are three premorbid (preceding the disorder) personality types which represent etiological qualities in alcoholism: the emotionally insecure, anxious, and dependent; the depressed; and the sociopath. He goes on to suggest the pre-alcoholic is "passive-dependent, egocentric, latently homosexual, a sociopath, intolerant of psychic tension, lacking in self-esteem and frightened of intimacy (p. 75)."

Vaillant (1995) summarizes four factors: culture, heredity, childhood, and premorbid personality in an effort to reduce the number of variables that will explain addiction. He uses multiple regression analysis, a statistical technique that estimates the relationship between interrelated predictor variables. Vaillant (1995) states it is a "crude approximation, which can suggest but never prove causation (p. 115)."

Vaillant goes on to say that no single set of traits determines alcoholism. Furthermore, a sociological model and a medical model can define it.

Vaillant's research is based on longitudinal studies. His first book looks at studies of men age 50, and this one follows up for the next 15 years. Most studies reflect a "snapshot" in time whereas a longitudinal study is like a "motion picture" (R. C. Madsen PhD, personal communication, January 10, 2006). Generally speaking, longitudinal studies may be more valid.

Comment for the Reader: Well, after this section you might conclude that there are more questions about an addictive personality than answers. Ha! You would be right! But the information is useful; it all has a certain flavor that describes the addict/alcoholic as at least and at best, as having certain vulnerabilities that cause them to react to drugs differently than others. These vulnerabilities are personality related. Personality is chemically (genetic/physiological) related. These vulnerabilities cause distress, dysfunction, and impairment.

CHAPTER 3

DISEASE MODEL

Some professions in the field believe addiction is a disease; some believe it is like a disease (Shaffer, 1990). Nowhere is there a comprehensive definition of what is meant that addiction is a disease. In essence, however, it seems to convey the notion that one may have little control over its onset; i.e., like diabetes. Also, while one cannot cure it, it is treatable. Inherent in this discussion is the role of responsibility – one may not bear the responsibility for being addictive – one is accountable for their recovery (Alcoholics Anonymous, 1976).

Although the disease model suggests etiology, it is more practically used as a treatment matrix and gives it form (Shaffer, 1990). Etiology is ambiguous and the disease model today also incorporates socio-cultural factors. Regardless, the medical model remains the dominant theory in the field (Peele, 1984). While treatment modalities have broadened, underlying theory has not changed all that much. The same concepts are in play: biological, genetic, and hereditary; psychological and personality theories; and socio-cultural and environmental.

The Diagnostic Statistical Manual (DSM-IV-TR), considered by most practitioners to be the psychiatric 'bible,' represents practical application in diagnosing substance abuse disorders. It characterizes substance dependence with 7 criteria. If three are met, describing a maladaptive pattern of substance use leading to clinical impairment in a 12-month period, there is chemical dependency.

DSM-IV

The DSM-IV (2004) has developed criteria to define substance dependence. It is referred to as "a cluster of cognitive, behavioral, and physiological symptoms (p. 192)." A diagnosis includes three of the following:

1) Tolerance – the need to use more to get the same effect.
2) Withdrawal – going through a withdrawal syndrome or using more substance to avoid it.
3) Taking the substance in greater amounts for a longer period than was intended.
4) Having a persistent desire or tried unsuccessful efforts to cut down or control the substance.
5) Great deal of time is spent getting the substance, using it, and recovering from its effects.
6) Missing social, occupational, or recreational activities in order to use substances.
7) Continuing to use despite knowledge of negative consequences.

Items 1, 2, and 3 are physiological factors. Eysenck's dopamine theory could fit this description. Items 4, 5, and 6 are behavioral factors. These items fit in with the psychoticism dimension. Item 7 is a cognitive factor. This fits in with the neuroticism dimension. Thus, proponents of an addictive personality are not in conflict with DSM-IV criteria for substance dependence.

> *Comment for the Reader:* As a substance abuse counselor in a community substance abuse agency, the writer provided individual and group counseling on an outpatient basis. In an Intensive Outpatient Program, which meets three times a week for four hours an evening, the writer provided psycho-education.

The psycho education part of the program is aimed at relapse prevention and this takes many forms. Drug education, 12-Step Program Orientation, Rational Recovery concepts, faith-based recovery, and peer-based recovery are included as well as providing insight into triggers for alcohol/drug use and coping skills for abstinence.

Triggers and coping skills rely on gleaned (if not proven) data regarding the addictive personality. The following is a list of triggers drawn up by 10 substance abuse clients in a recent psycho education group.

> Clients stated they frequently used drugs/alcohol when they were: worried, afraid, sad, depressed, frightened, fearful, anxious, lonely, bored, upset over a relationship, upset by an argument, angry, happy, feeling guilty, feeling ashamed, feeling impulsive, celebrating an accomplishment, lacking confidence, having a bad day, moody over a rainy day, excited about a warm and sunny day, having fun, socializing, done with work, waking up, going to sleep . . . the list, of course, could be endless.

It reflects, however, all the generalities we make about the addictive personality. It is high on neuroticism (negative emotionality) and psychoticism, and low on extraversion.

In my local recovery circle, two very interesting factors emerged. First, 80% of us were on some type of anti-depressant, anti-anxiety, or anti-psychotic medication or some combination thereof. Could Eysenck's references to the dopamine theory suggest addicts/alcoholics may have decreased dopamine levels? What are the implications for serotonin- and dopamine-related chemical therapy for the addict/alcoholic (Greenshaw, 2003)?

Again, the concept of the addict/alcoholic having a chemical imbalance is not a new one. The second item to emerge for this recovery circle is the notion of being "less than" (chemically related?). This refers to a certain feeling that many addicts/alcoholics relate to; that is, having an unfillable "hole in my soul" as one of my clients stated. Being "less than" is, not ever feeling good enough or not fitting in, as though one were deficient and/or inadequate.

There are a couple more things I want to mention in this section. Many of these characteristics we have described regarding an addictive personality fit in with diagnosing a co-occurring disorder, whether it be anxiety, depression, a personality disorder NOS (not otherwise specified), or some other mental health issue. Worthy of mention because it can be easily understood that an addictive personality, or let's just say one with a propensity for addiction, would go hand in hand with a co-occurring disorder, if not the basis for it. The concept of an addictive personality falls under psychological theories of addiction. It compliments the biological, medical model, disease concept. They fit together well. In other words, that "X" factor we spoke of at the beginning of the unit is no doubt a genetic factor. But, according to Eysenck (1991), it need not be a genetic factor. (No confusion here; he is just acknowledging that there are other factors involved.) He theorizes that even if our propensity is a learned phenomenon; i.e., socio-cultural, learning, or environmental, it becomes "hardwired" as though it was a genetic factor. Imagine that!

Motif in Drug Usage

Inaba and Cohen (2000) identify five reoccurring motives of drug use that emerge as we study the field. First of all, human beings have always struggled and contended with their environment and being, and have had a basic necessity to deal effectively with it. I think this is such a profound statement and concept. It implies, I believe, that one's desire to change one's consciousness is neither pathological nor blame-worthy. Second, the brain is inherently sensitive to psychoactive drugs. This is why people get into trouble with them. In other words, existence can be inherently strident and humans have always sought solace physically and psychologically. It makes it seem like a normal thing to do. It supports the idea that alcoholics/addicts are not responsible for being that way; only responsible to do something about it. Third, there is both government and private components involved with manufacturing and taxing drugs. Fourth, there have been significant technological improvements in manufacturing drugs. Lastly, there are new and faster ways to absorb chemicals into the body. These factors combine to form a pattern that propels drug usage today.

CHAPTER 4

History of Drug Usage, Treatment, and Recovery

History of Drug Usage. Inaba and Cohen (2000) provide a brief history of psychoactive drugs dated back to circa 5000 BC when certain plants were accidently discovered to have mood-altering properties, and then used for those purposes. Around early BC/AD, ancient cultures, such as the Egyptians, Chinese, South Americans, and others used opium, alcohol, cannabis, and psychedelics. During the middle ages, psychoactive plants were used by medicine men and the like, for cures to illnesses and for spiritual purposes. Around 1500, coffee, tea, alcohol, and opium production and consumption spread worldwide. Increased trade routes, expanded drug production, changing social customs, as well as increased legal and illegal drug usage characterized the 20th century. The medical model of addiction emerged and treatment developed. Drugs have affected the social, political and economic aspects of society. Inaba and Cohen (2000) state that drugs of choice change, but reasons why people use drugs stay the same.

History of Drug Treatment and Recovery

White (1998) provides a comprehensive history of Drug Treatment and Recovery. I will highlight it herein. It is interesting to note the various trends throughout history: moral, medical, and legal, which significantly impacted the way addicts/alcoholics were thought of and treated.

1700s. The first article on alcoholism known to be written was published by Anthony Benezet and was called *Mighty Destroyer Displayed.* In the same era, Native Americans formed sobriety "Circles" in order to provide support to each other. These "Circles" became incorporated into cultural renewal programs. Benjamin Rush, MD wrote *Inquiry into the Effects of Ardent Spirits on the Human Mind and Body,* which documented chronic drinking and contended that it is a disease and needed to be treated medically. This was the start of the American temperance movement. Prior to Rush's work, there was little awareness or concern regarding alcohol-related consequences.

1800s. In the early 1800s, Dr Rush started the first "Sober House." The Reverend Lyman Beecher wrote *Six Sermons On Intemperance* which described drinking as sin, stating that it became uncontrollable and provided warning signs of out-of-control drinking. Dr Samuel Woodward pointed to the need for asylums to care for drunkards. In the mid 1800s, The Washingtonian Society, a half million strong, evolved into the Fraternal Temperance Society, which in part was devoted to 'reforming' drinkers. Various Lodging Homes and a Home for the Fallen opened in Boston. Frederick Douglas, a self-disclosed former drinker, advocated for abstinence with African American people. He supported the abolition of slavery, as well as full citizenship based on principles of abstinence. This set the stage for African American models of sobriety. Magnus Huss, a physician from Sweden, wrote about a disease that ensues from chronic drinking. He called it *"Alcoholismus Chronicus."* The term 'alcoholism' emerged as a result. In the latter 1800s, The New York State Inebriate Asylum opened in Binghamton. It was the first of a number of institutions that would treat alcoholism and addiction to other drugs, such as opium, morphine, cocaine, chloral, ether, and chloroform. The Martha Washington Home in Chicago was the first facility that specialized in treating women. The American Association for the Cure of Inebriety publishes the *Journal of Inebriety* based on the premise that alcoholism was a disease. The Ribbon Reform Clubs began in the Northeast and spread nationwide. These were alcoholic groups that wore colored ribbons so that members could identify each other and convey a message of hope and recovery. Religious conversion became a hallmark remedy for alcoholism. Jerry McAuley started the Water Street Mission in New York City, and the Salvation Army further developed the first of an urban mission movement. The missions gave birth to mutual aid societies like the United Order of Ex-Boozers. The Salvation Army pursued the alcoholic cause with vigor, believing the only salvation was through Jesus Christ. The Salvation Army remains today to be one of the most unconditionally generous organizations to the care and well being of the alcoholic. Dr Leslie Keeley opened 120 Keeley Institutes across the country. Keeley believed that he could cure alcoholism. They were the first private for profit facilities in the United States. Keeley started a mail-order business that sold Double Chloride of Gold that was believed to cure tobacco and alcohol addictions. Dr Sigmund Freud and other physicians recommended cocaine for the treatment of alcoholism and morphine addiction. Hawkers sold bottled cures for alcoholism and drug addiction; they were later found to contain alcohol, opium, morphine, cocaine, and cannabis. The Keeley League was founded which advocated for medical treatment reform for the alcoholic as opposed to legal retorts. The roots of addiction medicine and recovery efforts began in the 1800s as did an increase in drug/alcohol use. Various methods of 'curing' alcoholism were attempted from 1840-1950. "Eugenics" was an attempt to eliminate alcoholism by genetically removing the gene pool for alcoholism; sterilization was believed to be the means of relieving future generations. Natural therapeutics was tried in the belief that a vegetarian diet could lead to sobriety. Water cures were attempted to wean alcoholics off liquor by watering down the alcohol. For a while, research was aimed at developing an alcoholism vaccine. Morphine was used to get people off alcohol; of course, what was considered reformation was actually drug substitution.

1900s. Treatment approaches continued to develop further throughout the 20th century both to alcohol and to narcotics and other drugs. Alcoholics Anonymous emerged into a type of movement. The Minnesota Model of treating alcoholism and drug addiction became the paradigm and is still most prevalent today.

In the early 1900s, inebriate homes and asylums closed, alcoholics wound up in "drunk tanks" in jail and "foul wards" in hospitals and the back wards of "insane asylums." Those with money sought private detoxification in private facilities known as "jitter joints," "jag farms," or "dip shops." The Charles B. Towns Hospital for Drug and Alcoholic Addictions opened in New York City and was the first of a new type of hospital for wealthy addicts and alcoholics. The Emmanuel Clinic in Boston began providing 'therapy' for the alcoholic, which became influential in the treatment of alcoholism for years to come. State laws emerged mandating treatment for "defectives;" the mentally ill, the developmentally disabled, and alcoholics and addicts. The Harrison Tax Act gave government control of opiates and cocaine accessible by physicians. Webb vs. the United States found that it is illegal medical practice for physicians to maintain patients' addiction, and some 25,000 doctors are indicted. Morphine Maintenance clinics opened by municipalities, but are eventually closed. Only the very wealthy were able to obtain treatment for narcotic addiction. In the 1920s, there was a collapse of Sober Houses, asylums, private institutions, and publications advocating the treatment of alcoholism.

Then in 1935, the Shadel Sanatorium began the use of classical aversive conditioning in a hospital treatment setting. "Narcotics Farms" opened in Lexington, KY, and in Fort Worth, TX, and the government began to get involved in addiction research and treatment. Also in 1935, Bill W. and Dr Bob met and began the formation of Alcoholics Anonymous (see chapter 5). In 1939, they published the book *Alcoholics Anonymous*. Soon after, the *Quarterly Journal of Studies on Alcohol* was published. Recovering alcoholics are hired by modern industry to form programs to aid the alcoholic. This later developed into employee assistance programs. Hypnosis became a primary method of treatment and is used off and on through the 1950's.

In 1941, The *Saturday Evening Post* published an article about Alcoholics Anonymous and AA growth was rapid and widespread. Public education is elicited to change Americans' views of the alcoholic. Yale initiated significant research programs. In 1944, The National Committee for Education on Alcoholism was founded on five premises, which mirrored the disease concept and AA practices. The first premise was that alcoholism is a disease. Secondly, this implied that the alcoholic was a sick person. The third premise was that the alcoholic can be helped. Fourth, the alcoholic was worth helping. And fifth, alcoholism was the #4 public health problem and had become the responsibility of society to remedy. The committee is known today as The National Council on Alcoholism and Drug Dependence. In the 1950s, there were attempts at controlled drinking research, which was and still is a controversial and provocative issue.

In the mid-1900s, state alcoholism commissions were developed; they supported treatment and education efforts at the community level. Addicts Anonymous began in Lexington, KY. In New York, it was called Narcotics Anonymous, but didn't last. Today's NA began in groups based in CA around 1953. Alcoholics Victorious, a Christian recovery support group was formed in Chicago and was favored in many city missions. The "Minnesota Model" of treatment emerged and looked a lot like many programs today, including evaluation, intake, treatment planning, therapeutic counseling, and discharge planning. The "Minnesota Model" is based on AA philosophy. The use of Disulfram (antabuse) becomes the predominant method of treatment. In 1950, the 12 Traditions were incorporated into AA. AA membership was around 100,000 and the country became interested in alcoholism. Hollywood came out with many classic films, such as *Days of Wine and Roses*. The Association of Halfway House Alcoholism Programs of North America was founded in 1958 following a halfway house movement. In 1951, Al-Anon emerged from the rise of Family Groups started by Lois W. and Anne B. In 1952, the American Medical Association defines alcoholism. In 1954, R. Brinkley Smithers, a self-disclosed recovering alcoholic and participant in the Yale Summer School of Alcohol Studies, raised $37 million for research and education. The American Society of Addiction Medicine (ASAM) was founded and was the first agency to approve state jobs for alcohol counselors. In 1957, the Veteran's Administration began treating alcoholism and the American Hospitals Association resolved to end discrimination against alcoholics. In 1958, Charles Dederich, a recovering addict, found Synanon, which became a model for drug treatment programs in the 1960s and 1970s.

In 1960, E. M. Jellinek published *The Disease Concept of Alcoholism*. This is still considered today to be a seminal work in the medical (disease) model of addiction. In 1961, the American Bar Association and the American Medical Association published a report, *Drug Addiction: Crime or Disease?* and advocated for community-based treatment programs. In 1963, The American Public Health Association identified alcoholism as a treatable illness. In the mid-60s federal funding increased and supported local alcohol and addiction treatment programs. Also, Dr Vincent Dole and Dr Marie Nyswander introduced methadonetherapy.

In the early 1970s, insurance companies began to reimburse for treatment. This created significant growth in private and hospital-based programs. In 1965, the American Psychiatric Association encouraged its doctors to learn about alcoholism and encouraged insurance companies to cover alcoholism treatment. Also, two Federal Court decisions upheld the disease concept of alcoholism and President Johnson stated that the disease would yield to research and treatment. In 1971, the American Journal of Psychiatry published *Criteria for the Diagnosis of Alcoholism*. In 1972, the Joint Commission on Accreditation of Hospitals developed standards for alcoholism treatment. The Food and Drug Administration approved methadone for treating heroin addiction. Vernon Johnson's book, *I'll Quit Tomorrow*, introduced methods to treat alcoholics before they "hit bottom" which was originally believed to be a prerequisite to recovery. In the mid 70s, credentialing for alcohol counselors began. There were controversies over whether alcoholism and drug abuse treatment should be integrated (which did not begin to occur until the 1980s). In 1978, Betty Ford, the President's wife announced that she entered recovery from alcohol and other drugs.

Mothers Against Drunk Driving was formed in 1980. In 1981, Nancy Reagan initiated the "Just Say No" campaign which began a "zero tolerance" approach to drug usage. This decreased federal support from treatment programs and increased the number of drug users incarcerated. As a result, drug courts developed and treatment programs began in prisons in the 1990s. Cocaine Anonymous began in 1982. The legal drinking age was raised to 21 in 1984. Crack cocaine was introduced in the mid '80s. In the late '80s, increasing concern emerged for special populations including women, adolescents, the elderly, gays and lesbians, and the 'dually diagnosed.' In 1987, President Reagan renewed the "War on Drugs" and there was a continued shift from treatment to punishment. At the same time, certain harm reduction practices took hold; i.e., needle exchange programs (see chapter 6). The American Medical Association, nonetheless, endorsed drug dependency treatment as a legitimate medical practice. In 1989, Stanton Peele published *Diseasing of America: Addiction Treatment Out of Control* and began an advocacy whose main mission was the opposition of 12-Step programs and treatment.

In the early 1990s, managed insurance care was aggressively implemented and alcoholism treatment was downsized, and a trend toward the integration of psychiatric treatment and substance abuse treatment began. It was called Behavioral Health Services and leaned toward outpatient services, instead of inpatient hospitalizations. In the 1990s, as a result of the Internet, there was large growth seen of recovery groups, services, education, and information available to all. The American Society of Addiction Medicine (ASAM) criteria shifted treatment to a level-of-care system based upon basic criteria of risk and severity of drug use, and consequence potential. In the mid 90s, there was a resurgence of poly-drug usage among the young and adolescent treatment approaches emerged. In 1995, the Food and Drug Administration approved naltrexone for treating alcoholism and other drug addictions.

2000s. In the *Journal of the American Medical Association* (McLellan, Lewis, O'Brien, & Kleber, 2000) recommended reconceptualizing addiction as a chronic medical illness and the disease model continued to predominate. In the early 21st century, there has been an increasing trend toward integrated dual diagnosis treatment. Unit 5 provides a description of the history of integrated dual diagnosis treatment.

Comment for the Reader: This stuff is interesting if you're into history. Probably what's important to know is that attitudes toward addiction/alcoholism and addicts/alcoholics fluctuated over the years, creating trends in treatment. It is unclear whether attitudes were dictated by moral, medical, and legal edicts or vice versa!

CHAPTER 5

HISTORY OF ALCOHOLICS ANONYMOUS

Cheever (2005), Wilson (1997), and AA (*Alcoholics Anonymous Comes of Age*) provide ample history regarding the life of Bill Wilson and the development of Alcoholics Anonymous. The story is highlighted here. Bill Wilson and Dr Bob Smith are credited with the organization of Alcoholics Anonymous. Bill W. was a financier, whose career collapsed due to his drinking. In 1934, he went into treatment with Dr William Silkworth. Silkworth was director of the Charles B. Towns Hospital for Drug/Alcohol Addictions in New York City and supported the disease concept of alcoholism. He helped Bill W. to understand that alcoholism was not just a moral issue but that it had a medical basis. Bill W. was admitted three times following relapses. Bill had a friend that he used to drink with, Edwin Throckmorton (Ebby) Thacher, who introduced him to spiritual principles he had learned while studying with the Oxford Group, as well as some Jungian theories.

Rowland Hazard III was a patient of Carl Jung who believed that alcoholism was a hopeless condition, and required spiritual experience in order to recover. During Hazard's spiritual quest, he joined the Oxford Group and subsequently became friends with Ebby Thacher. The Oxford Group, a Christian Fellowship, was popular for a brief time around 1925. It emphasized that sin was central to the human experience and surrender to God was the only solution. Sharing one's experiences with each other was vital; group consensus was critical and life sustaining. Wilson is said to have stopped drinking and turned to God. But the desire to drink returned and he sought help with Dr Bob Smith, who was also struggling. The two decided that working with other alcoholics is what kept them sober, and co-founded AA. Dr Bob is said to have had his last drink on June 10, 1935, which became the anniversary of AA. Within two years, the two had reached out to over 100 alcoholics. With the help of other members, Wilson published *Alcoholics Anonymous* in 1939, which became known as the *"Big Book."* It contained the 12 Steps which, in a July 1953 edition of the AA *Grapevine,* Bill W. indicated they were inspired by the Oxford Group's, Dr William Silkworth and psychologist William James.

The Oxford Group believed in a type of confession called "sharing," practiced making amends, and was based on complete honesty. They sought guidance from God through 'quiet times.' Ebby and Bill talked about being 'released' from the desire to drink as opposed to needing to fight the desire to drink. Dr Silkworth had been proclaiming for years that alcoholism was an illness. While in the hospital, Bill had been brought a copy of William James' book, *Varieties of Religious Experience.* James believed that spirituality made people function more effectively, and furthermore thoroughly and dramatically changed people into becoming able to do things they had otherwise been unable to do and had not thought possible.

When writing the Big Book, the first four chapters were collaboratively drafted with great exuberance. Chapter Five needed to actually explain what the program was and determined that a set of principles (eventually called the steps) spelling things out clearly was necessary.

In 30 minutes, Bill started with:

1. We admitted that we were powerless over alcohol.
2. We got honest with ourselves.
3. We got honest with another person, in confidence.
4. We made amends for harm done to others.
5. We worked with other alcoholics without demand for prestige or money.
6. We prayed to God to help us do these things as best we could.

When it was presented to the New York meeting, there was much protest and discussion that went on for days. Agnostic supporters, Hank P. and Jim B. advocated for such language as "a Higher Power" and "God as we understand him" in an effort to reach the greatest numbers possible and without excluding people. Six steps developed into twelve and there was consensus. Furthermore, they received non-denominational support and support from the medical profession as well.

Due to publicity, religious, and financial conflicts and issues, the Twelve Traditions, first known as Twelve Points to Assure our Future, emerged in 1950. In 1955, at the Alcoholics Anonymous St. Louis, Missouri convention, Bill Wilson turned the guidance and direction of Alcoholics Anonymous over to the General Service Conference.

Comment for the Reader: At some point, every recovering person in 12-step programs enjoys knowing the history of AA, as the early roots set the stage for what the fellowship of the program is like today.

CHAPTER 6

Harm Reduction Theory (Harm Reduction: Recovery Reduction?)

To this point, history and addiction theories have supported the concept of complete abstinence from all chemical substances as the goal of addiction treatment. Seemingly contrary to this concept is the harm reduction theory (MacMaster, 2004). Harm reduction theory in treatment planning contradicts disease model traditional treatment planning of complete and total abstinence. Harm reduction goals are aimed at reducing the use of alcohol and other drugs and/or reducing the harm related to alcohol and other drug use. Examples of these are methadone programs and needle exchange programs (MacMaster, 2004). Along the lines of harm reduction, controlled drinking is another alternative perspective, which supports the notion that different kinds of alcohol/drug problems require different kinds of responses (Ambrogne, 2002; Humphreys, 2003; Polich, Armor, & Braiker, 1981). Polich, Armor and Braiker (1981) research suggested that 18% of clients described problem-free drinking four years post treatment. Harm reduction is probably more an approach to substance abuse treatment than an addiction theory, but it is placed in this first unit for two reasons. First of all, not everyone walking in the doors of treatment has an addiction issue. Secondly, abstinence as the primary goal, may not always be effective. So it is a departure from the traditional concept of recovery – and a confusing one.

Harm reduction, simply put, is putting focus on reducing drug-related harm vs. reducing drug use. It was originally suggested in England in the 1920s as part of the Rolleston Committee's recommendations concerning drug use. It emerged again in the 1980s in response to a rise in hepatitis C. In several Western Europe countries, it is the basis for drug policy; it has also been the foundation for policy in the Netherlands for over 30 years. The Dutch have used harm reduction since the early 1970s. Harm reduction theory has been used in Switzerland and Germany as well. These are examples of macro system influences. In the United States, in the 1960s, methadone maintenance programs began in an effort to reduce drug-related crime, and provide a solution to heroin addiction. Recently, the United States has begun using these theories in response to the increased spread of AIDS. Needle exchange programs have emerged in a few major cities in an effort to reduce illness resulting from dirty needles (MacMaster, 2004). Providing these services for clients is at a micro level. Drug related harm (drug usage, drug-related crime, and drug-related health issues) rose to catastrophic proportions. Methadone and needle exchange serve as historical reference points in substance abuse treatment.

"The preventable harm caused by HIV/AIDS clearly outweighs the need to adhere to the abstinence-based perspective. Quite simply, dead addicts don't recover"(MacMaster, 2004, p. 360).Don't you love that? It's a good point, right? So, although many of us cringe at the thought of the harm reduction theory; there is a time and place for it.

Alcoholics Anonymous (AA) is the basis for abstinence theory and 12-step programs as well. It emerged in the 1940s (inception 6/10/35) through the efforts of Bill Wilson and Dr Bob. It is a fellowship that focuses on meetings, 12 steps, and belief in a higher power. The 12 steps is a program of change. Alcoholics acknowledge their illness and unmanageability, go through lifestyle, behavioral, and cognitive changes ideally culminating in a psychic change or spiritual awakening. (Alcoholics Anonymous, 1976). Other 12-step programs have emerged since: for drugs (narcotics) = NA, for cocaine = CA, for gambling = GA, for sexual addictions = SA. AA is also a macro systems approach to crisis intervention.

Harm reduction strategies, combined with conventional abstinence-based theories, can provide a foundation for working with individuals with substance abuse problems (MacMaster, 2004). However, caregivers must understand both perspectives and their client's level of motivation for change, and use the model that best suits the situation.

Harm reduction theories embrace certain key concepts. They seek to reduce the amount of harm-related consequences to drug use; i.e., physical, emotional, legal, familial, unemployment, etc., without necessarily eliminating the drug use. There can be different approaches. People can be discouraged from using drugs. This is known as prevalence reduction. People can be encouraged to reduce the amount and/or the frequency of their usage. This is quantity reduction. We can also try to reduce the negative consequences from drug use. This is known as harm reduction. Usually these approaches are integrated (MacCoun, 1998).

According to MacMaster (2004), drugs are a part of our world. As a result, it makes more sense to focus 'on reducing drug-related harm than reducing drug use' (p. 359).

Comment for the Reader: How do you feel about that? Abstinence from drug usage, clearly effective, is seen as only one way to reduce substance-related harm. MacMaster (2004) states that many of the more serious consequences of drug use; i.e., HIV/AIDS, hepatitis, overdoses, car accidents, etc., can be reduced without complete abstinence. Harm reduction approaches are praised for meeting the consumer where he is. Subsequently, services must be relevant and meet the consumer's choice of the direction of treatment if they are to be effective.

In a conversation with Wayne Trudeau, executive operations analyst for the State of Connecticut's Department of Mental Health and Addiction Services, who assisted in the creation of, approval, and implementation of programs in the state, Mr. Trudeau stated "Abstinence is good, but you don't get many takers."

MacMaster (2004) purports that we, as a society, will always be afflicted by disease and related social problems. The harm-reduction approach utilizes the human service model. It expects drug abuse to be prevalent, creating social problems that will continue to affect clients' lives.

This writer's concern is that in an effort to meet the consumer where he is, clinicians are becoming conditioned to settle for less than abstinence – as a goal in treatment. This sends the message that substance usage is tacitly approved of. When clinicians are taught, for example, that relapse is part of the process as purported by harm-reduction advocates; this writer believes that this gets conveyed on some level to the consumer.

This can be a dangerous practice. Drug addicts typically, can lead a dangerous lifestyle while obtaining, using, and being high on drugs. The clinician cannot let this go without addressing it. Core ethical principles of non-maleficence (do no harm) and beneficence (client welfare first) are subject here (Herlihy & Corey, 1996). Clearly both harm-reduction strategies and abstinence programs have their pluses and minuses. It is important to meet the client where he is or you may lose the person altogether. It is important to at least keep the door open for future dialogue. At the very minimum, the harm-reduction approach does what it can to keep the addict alive long enough to decide to stop using.

The clinician must be well-versed on both harm reduction and abstinence approaches. He must know his client well. And he must be adept at combining both approaches. If the client opts not to attend a 12-Step Program, the clinician must aid the client in a sustaining means of recovery. Some people achieve abstinence thru AA. Some turn to spirituality and/or religion. Some have a revelation. Some gain it through psychotherapy, through solution-focused skills, through medication or a combination of any of these methods (more in unit 7). But there must be something ongoing and ever-present that has changed if a person is to avoid drinking/drugging again.

> *Comment for the Reader:* Harm reduction is useful and realistic, don't dismiss it. Yes, I do know it can be dangerous information in the wrong hands! It's realistic because 1) recovery is a process and you have to start somewhere, and 2) you will lose people if you shove abstinence down their throat. It is dangerous because it is misleading. Ultimately abstinence should be the goal for any chemically dependent person and the counselor needs to be able to at least point things in that direction when working collaboratively with the client without turning him off.

And remember, we are talking about the chemically *dependent* person. There are those that come into our offices because they have gotten into trouble – which may be situational. It does not necessarily mean they are dependent. I always direct the clients to answer this question for themselves: "can I drink/drug safely?" And that answer is a relative thing!

Conclusion

The goal of this unit is to help create a foundation for how substance abuse is approached in the field today and it's my hope that you have some food for thought as you may formulate and further develop your own perspectives for treatment and recovery. The next unit will shift to present an overview of counseling theory in practice today. It is intended to provide background for your theoretical approach to counseling.

UNIT 1 Highlights

CH 1/Addiction Theory

- Biological Theory = Medical Model/Disease Concept/ Genetic Theory
- Psychological Theory = Addictive Personality
- Behavior Theory = Addiction is learned/not a disease

CH 2/The Addictive Personality

- There are too many factors with too many variables to research addictive personality empirically
- Much data gathered
- Addicts/alcoholics have an "X" factor
- Addiction/alcoholism correlated with introversion, instability, anti-social, emotionality, impulsivity, reward dependence, novelty seeking, harm avoidance, low frustration level, helplessness, and more
- Is the addict/alcoholic precipitated by personality type?
- Is the addict/alcoholic personality type the result of drinking/drugging?

CH 3/Disease Model

- Is addiction/alcoholism a disease? Or is it like a disease?
- Provides conceptual etiology for addiction/alcoholism
- Provides foundation for treatment planning
- Removes self-blame/responsibility for being addict/alcoholic

CH 4/History of Drug Use, Treatment, and Recovery

- Man has always contended with his environment and being, and sought means to cope with it
- 1700s: Recognition of alcoholic/problematic drinking/Temperance Movement begins
- 1800s: Various sober houses and treatment modalities emerge; i.e., eugenics, natural therapeutics, water cures, morphine
- 1900s: Treatment develops/Disease concept popular/Minnesota Program Model/Alcoholics Anonymous founded and expanded/Mothers Against Drunk Drivers founded and expanded/U.S. Commissions funded/punishment vs. treatment modes vacillate.
- 2000s: Integrated Dual Diagnosis Treatment is the new paradigm along with person-centered theory recovery core values

CH 5/History of Alcoholics Anonymous

- 1935/Bill W. enters treatment
- Bill W. and Dr Bob found AA with the influence of Dr Silkworth, William James, the Oxford Movement, and Carl Jung, and they write the *Big Book*
- 1950/12 Traditions added
- 1955/General Service Office founded
- 1960 to the present/AA flourishes and expands worldwide

CH 6/Harm Reduction Theory

- Harm reduction or recovery reduction?
- 1) Reduce harm related to substance use 2) reduce frequency of use 3) discourage use

Study Guide

1) Which theory of addiction hits home with you? Why?
2) Do you support the concept of an addictive personality? Why? Why not?
3) Do you feel the Harm Reduction Approach is viable? Why? Why Not?

References

Ait-Daoud, N.; Roache, J.; Dawes, M.; Liu, L.; Wang, X.; Javors, M, et al. (2009). Can serotonin transporter genotype predict craving in alcoholism? *Alcoholism: Clinical and Experimental Research,* 33(8), 1329-1335. doi:10.1111/j.1530-0277.2009.00962.x.

Alcoholics Anonymous (1939). *Alcoholics Anonymous.* Alcoholics Anonymous World Services.

Alcoholics Anonymous (3rd ed.) (1976). NY: Alcoholics Anonymous World Services, Inc.

Ambrogne, J. (2002). Reduced-risk drinking as a treatment goal: What clinicians need to know. *Journal of Substance Abuse Treatment,* 22(1), 45-53. doi:10.1016/S0740-5472(01)00210-0.

Andres-Hyman, R. (2004, December). Recovery Core Values. Handout Presented at Connecticut Department of Mental Health and Addiction Services Education and Training, Hartford CT.

American Psychiatric Association. (2004). *Diagnostic and Statistical Manual* – IV-TR. American Psychiatric Association.

Cheever, S. (2005). *My name is Bill W.* NY, NY: Washington Square Press

Connecticut Certification Board, Inc. *Alcoholism and Substance Abuse Counselors' Code of Ethics.* [Electronic Version]. Retrieved 4/29/05.

Corey, G. (2009). *Theory and practice of counseling and psychotherapy* (8th ed.). Belmont, CA: Brooks/Cole.

Davis, D.R. & Jansen, G.G. (1998). Making meaning of alcoholics anonymous for social workers: myths, metaphors, and realities. [Electronic Version] *Social Work,* 43(2), 169-182.

Eysenck, H. J. (1991). Neuroticism, anxiety, and depression. [Electronic Version]. *Psychological Inquiry,* 2(1), 75-77.

Eysenck, H. J. (1997). Addiction, personality and motivation. [Electronic Version] *Human Psychopharmacology, Clinical and Experimental,* 12(2), 79-87.

Gossop, M. R. & Eysenck, S. B. G. (1980). A further investigation into the personality of drug addicts in treatment. [Electronic Version] *British Journal of Addiction,* 75, 305-311.

Greenshaw, A. J. (2003). Neurotransmitter interactions in psychotropic drug action: beyond dopamine and serotonin. [Electronic Version] *Psychiatry Nuerosci,* 28(4), 247-250.

Hendriks, V. M. (1990). Psychiatric disorders in a Dutch addict population: rates and correlates of DSM-III diagnosis. [Electronic Version] *Journal of Consulting and Clinical Psychology,* 58(2), 158-165.

Herlihy, B., Corey, G. (1996). *ACA Ethical Standards Casebook.* Alexandria, VA: American Counseling Association.

Humphreys, K. (2003). Alcoholics Anonymous and 12-step alcoholism treatment programs. Recent developments in alcoholism, Volume 16: Research on alcoholism treatment (pp. 149-164). New York, NY US: Kluwer Academic/Plenum Publishers. Retrieved from PsycINFO database.

Inaba, D.S.; Cohen, W.E. (2004). *Uppers, downers, all arounders: Physical and mental effects of psychoactive drugs* (5th ed.). Medford, OR: CNS Publications, Inc.

Jellinek, E.M. (1960). *The disease concept of alcoholism.* New Haven, CT: College Press.

Johnson, T. (2007). Cultural-level influences on substance use & misuse. *Substance Use & Misuse,* 42(2-3), 305-316. doi:10.1080/10826080601142022.

Kagan, D. M. (2001). Addictive personality factors. [Electronic Version] *The Journal of Psychology,* 121(6), 533-538.

Kerr, J. S. (1996). Two myths of addiction: the addictive personality and the issue of free choice. [Electronic Version] *Human Psychopharmacology,* II, 9-13.

Kinney, J., & Leaton, G. (1987). *Loosening the Grip: A Handbook of Alcohol Information* (3rd ed.). St Louis, MO: Times Mirror/ Mosby College Publishing.

Kurtz, E. (1991). *Not God: A history of alcoholics anonymous.* Center City, MN: Hazelden Pittman Archives Press.

Quintero, G.; Peterson, J.; & Young, B. (2006). An Exploratory Study of Socio-Cultural Factors Contributing to Prescription Drug Misuse Among College Students. *Journal of Drug Issues,* 36(4), 903-932. Retrieved from PsycINFO database.

Lawson, G.; Peterson, J.; & Lawson, A. (1983). *Alcoholism and the family.* Rockville, MD: Andover Press.

MacMaster, S.A. (2004). Harm reduction: a new perspective on substance abuse services. [Electronic version] *Social Work,* 49(3), 356-364.

MacCoun, R.J. (1998). Toward a psychology of harm reduction. [Electronic Version] *American Psychologist,* 53(11), 1199-1208.

McGue, M.; Slutske, W.; & Iacono, W. G. (1999). Personality and substance use disorders: II. Alcoholism versus drug use disorders. [Electronic Version] *Journal of Consulting and Clinical Psychology,* 67(3), 394-404.

Moos, R.H.; Moos, B.S. (2004). Long-term influence of duration and frequency of participation in alcoholics anonymous on individuals with alcohol use disorders. [Electronic version] *Journal of Consulting and Clinical Psychology,* 72(1), 81-90.

Mustanski, B. S.; Viken, R. J.; Kaprio, J.; & Rose, R. J. (2003). Genetic influences on the association between personality risk factors and alcohol. [Electronic Version] *Journal of Abnormal Psychology,* 112(2), 282-289.

Nathan, P.E. (1988). The addictive personality is the behavior of the addict. [Electronic Version] *Journal of Consulting and Clinical Psychology,* 56(2), 183-188.

Peele, Stanton. 1984. "The cultural context of psychological approaches to alcoholism: Can we control the effects of alcohol?" *American Psychologist* 39(12), 1337-1351. PsycARTICLES, EBSCOhost (accessed April 21, 2009).

Pervin, L.; Cervone, D.; & Oliver, J. (2005). *HS 814 theories of personality.* Hoboken, NJ: John Wiley and Sons, Inc.

Polich, J. Michael; Armor, David J.; Braiker, Harriet B. (1981). The Course of Alcoholism: Four Years After Treatment; New York: Wiley.

Prochaska, J.O.; Diclemente, C.C.; Norcross, J.C. (1992). In search of how people change: applications to addictive behaviors. [Electronic Version] *American Psychologist,* 47(9), 1102-1114.

Scherling, D.H. (2004, October). Hopeful Conversations: *Inspiring Recovery Through Motivational Interviewing.* Handout Presented at Connecticut Department of Mental Health and Addiction Services Education and Training, Middletown, CT.

Shaffer, H. (1990). Addictive disease in the nineties: Lessons from the emperor. *Psychology of Addictive Behaviors,* 4(1), 57-64.

Sher, K. J.; Bartholow, B. D.; & Wood, M. D. (2000). Personality and substance abuse disorders: a prospective study. [Electronic Version] *Journal of Consulting and Clinical Psychology,* 68(5), 818-829.

Sher, K. J.; & Trull, T. J. (1994). Personality and disinhibitory psychology: alcoholism and anti-social personality disorder. [Electronic Version] *Journal of Abnormal Psychology,* 103(1), 92-102.

Slutske, W. S.; Heath, A. C.; Madden, P. A.; Bucholz, K. K.; Statham, D. J.; & Martin, N. G. (2002). Personality and the genetic risk for alcohol dependence. [Electronic Version] *Journal of Abnormal Psychology,* 111(1), 124-133.

Sutker, P. B.; & Allain, A. N. (1988). Issues in personality conceptualizations of addictive behaviors. [Electronic Version] *Journal of Consulting and Clinical Psychology,* 56(2), 172-182.

Tarter, R. E. (1988). Are there inherited behavioral traits that predispose to substance abuse? [Electronic Version] *Journal of Consulting and Clinical Psychology,* 56(2), 189-196.

Twelve Steps and Twelve Traditions. (1985). NY: Alcoholics Anonymous World Services, Inc.

White, W. (1998). *Slaying the Dragon: The History of Addiction Treatment and Recovery in America.* Bloomington, IL: Chestnut Health Systems.

Wilson, B. (1997). *Pass it on.* NY, NY: Alcoholics Anonymous World Services.

Vaillant, G.E. (1995). *The Natural History of Alcoholism Revisited.* USA: Harvard College.

UNIT 2/Synopsis of Counseling Theories

Introduction

This unit shall present an overview of thematic concepts found in the more prevalent counseling theories utilized today. It is a broad-brush synopsis of several formal theories of therapy. The reader is referred to texts on personality theory or counseling theory for further in-depth explanations. The purpose is to demonstrate their applications in current substance abuse counseling in order to provide a background and a foundation for the counselor's counseling style. Many entry level substance abuse counselors might prefer to fly by the seat of their pants – and there is a time and place for that – but, as we will see by best practices, it is important to be grounded in theory as it provides a framework for working with your clients. Many counselors have good instincts, but it is important to know why you're doing what you're doing. It is hoped that you will see some of your ideas in action in the following descriptions and be able to put a name or theory to what you may be doing naturally.

There are generally considered to be three overall perspectives on therapy: these are psychoanalytic, humanistic, and behavioral. Psychoanalytical approaches include Sigmund Freud, Alfred Adler, Carl Jung, and others. Humanistic approaches include Carl Rogers, Frederick Perls, Rollo May, Victor Frankl, and others. Behavioral approaches include B.F. Skinner, Albert Ellis, William Glasser and others. Each offer useful contributions to substance use counseling. There are what is considered to be best practices and preferred methods of use today. The substance abuse counselor wants to have a menu of options in their repertoire. This represents an eclectic approach. An eclectic approach became a catchall phrase that covered an "anything goes" approach. An eclectic approach, however, is meant to be used with rhyme and reason to meet the clients needs, based on an understanding and an ability to apply various techniques.

Comment for the Reader: The new professional jargon is to say 'substance use' counseling as opposed to 'substance abuse' counseling . . . but, I can't get used to it. The point is that to say 'use' instead of 'abuse' reduces client stigma. What do you think?

CHAPTER 7

Psychodynamic Theory

Psychodynamic Theory: Corey (2009) explains that psychodynamic psychotherapy theorists include Sigmund Freud, Carl Jung, and Alfred Adler. There were many psychoanalytic revisionists (including Karen Horney, Eric Fromm, and Harry Stack Sullivan) and there were many theorists to come that were influenced by psychoanalytic theory (even if it was to reject it). The psychodynamic concept of human nature suggests that behavior is determined by internal forces: unconscious, instinctual, and biological (Corey, 2009). The term psychodynamic refers to the systemized psychological concepts, and the term psychoanalytic refers to its form of intensive therapy. The aim of psychoanalytic therapy is to make the unconscious conscious (Corey, 2009). Psychoanalytic theory implies that the root of all forms of neurosis and behavior is unconscious, and by bringing these motives and influences out, people can then exercise more choice in their decision-making (Corey, 2009).

Basically, there are two types of issues that people experience: conflict and crisis. Conflict refers to internal issues concerning unfinished business or unresolved personal issues. These issues are usually from the past; i.e., childhood abuse (physical, sexual, mental, or emotional), difficult relationships with parents, loss of a loved one, and so forth. Crisis tends to deal with here and now issues; i.e., divorce, loss of job, relationship difficulties, and so forth. Psychodynamic therapy deals with conflicts that are centered in the past. Certainly, conflicts can manifest themselves in crisis in the present, but their origins are from the past.

Sigmund Freud. Pervin et al. (2005) discuss Freud. Freud's theories revolve around the structure of the personality and its development. He suggests there is a conflict going on within us as a result of different forces. The id, or the pleasure motivated construct, seeks immediate gratification to avoid tension. The ego emerges in response to the id as a result of an inability to fulfill all of one's needs. The ego is based in reality. The superego begins to develop around age 5; it acts as the conscience, and deliberates between right and wrong based on the values learned from parents and the community.

Freud states that a conflict arises between the id and the ego and/or superego and creates anxiety. When the conflict is not resolved, one resorts to the usage of a variety of defense mechanisms that attempt to basically change the perception of reality on an unconscious level. While defense mechanisms help us cope, they may prevent the individual from resolving the anxiety and it may re-emerge.

Freud believed there are sexual drives originating with the id and that there are stages of development (oral, anal, phallic, latency, and genital). The lack of satisfactory gratification of sexual needs during these preset stages determines personality outcomes. Freud believed that our conflicts as adults are the result of these unmet needs. He used dream analysis and free association to uncover these unresolved unconscious issues.

There is one other important concept we gain from psychoanalytic therapy and that is the idea of transference and counter-transference. Transference is a complicated concept, which basically takes the place when the client projects emotions they have for a parent or significant other person onto the therapist. This can take many forms and may be the basis for trust and emotional dependence on the therapist. Counter-transference implies that the counselor is having emotional reactions to the client that may be relevant to the counselor's life.

Comment for the Reader: Substance abuse counseling today is more 'here and now' oriented. Counseling seems to focus more on skills, tools, and strategies that are solution focused. Psychoanalytic therapy is more interpretative. However, psychoanalytic therapy has had a major effect on the development of most fundamental theories of therapy. There are several useful concepts that the counselor can adapt into their repertoire of skills in substance use counseling. First is the notion that there are unconscious motives why people use substances. Some of these may be the result of unresolved issues in the past. It becomes, then, important to uncover what these underlying conflicts may be. This approach may not be applicable to all users as there are different reasons why people use, but it is a fundamental perspective with many clients. This approach to counseling is apt to come later in the recovery process. If the client was on a boat that was rapidly sinking, they shouldn't sit there and wonder why the boat is sinking. They need to get off the boat! Later, after finding safe harbor in recovery, the addict/alcoholic can begin to explore these other issues. Initial recovery skills, solution-focused and cognitive behavioral techniques will be described later in the text.

Corey (2009) tells us that unresolved anxiety leads to the natural and habitual inclination and tendency to use defense mechanisms. Isn't denial the biggest defense mechanism of all for the addict/alcoholic? All counselors are familiar with the fact that denial is a hallmark symptom of addiction/alcoholism. Denial prevents the addict/alcoholic from being dealt with and it continues to re-emerge.

Carl Jung broke with psychoanalytic theory on three major principles (Pervin et al., 2005; Corey, 2009). He did not believe that our conflicts were the result of sexual energy, but from a more generalized force in one's life. While he recognized the impact of the unconscious, he thought conflict was the result of one's hopes, plans, and dreams for the future or striving for self-actualization, and this is what produces anxiety. Lastly, Jung believed there was what he called the "collective unconscious." The individual can theoretically unconsciously tap into a reservoir of memory derived from the collective experiences of the human race. This is actually a metaphysical concept and suggests that people have an unconscious access to a universal mind. The field of psychology had difficulty with this concept, and it never became mainstream, though it did find its place in spiritual circles (LaChance, 2005).

Jung fostered the concept that one's goal in life is individuation; or reaching our goals and becoming all we can become (Pervin et al., 2005). This includes understanding one's unconscious processes as well as an integration of our thoughts, emotions, and intuition. Jung also used free association, dream analysis, symptom treatment, and the client's presentation of a life history (Corey, 2009).

> *Comment for the Reader:* Clearly one's frustration around unmet personal goals is a source of conflict for many people. Whether in the area of education, relationships, financial, professional and so forth, one's disappointments and failures, perceived or otherwise, create conflict and significantly impact one's self-esteem. Use of the life history serves to identify deficient patterns of behavior and generate a picture of how the client views his life. The life history is used in the 12 Steps of Alcoholics Anonymous (step 4) as well as narrative therapy (included later in this unit). Reframing the client's perception of their life history can modify the hues in the picture they possess of their lives.

Alfred Adler. Adler was also a disciple from Freud's theories, but parted ways in several areas (Pervin et al., 2005). Adler did not think the unconscious (especially sexually) plays as a significant role in one's behavior. Like Jung, he believed that future goals were more relevant than past history, and that people's lives are the result of their choices (Pervin et al., 2005; Corey, 2009). Adler thought that dysfunction arose in people's lives as a result of a mistaken perception of their lives (Corey, 2009). Corey (2009) explains further that Adler felt people developed feelings of inferiority, which held them back in their efforts to succeed. Like Freud, he thought early experiences were influential in people's lives and that social factors were very important; i.e., family of origin, birth order, family history, and social interests. He felt distorted impressions of one's life impacted on success. Adler thought dreams were important practice for future events. He often used role-play to help people adapt new skills. Adler felt people were often discouraged as opposed to being sick.

> *Comment for the Reader:* Certainly addiction/alcoholism involves obsession and compulsion and the writer does not think that one is responsible for having it, but rather one is accountable, nonetheless, for their behavior and is responsible for their recovery (as they say in the rooms). And so, when one is coming to terms with their addiction/alcoholism, there are choices that will be made. People's misperceptions over the past relate to what we stated about Adler's need to reframe the past. This concept is revisited when we discuss narrative therapy. In summary, psychodynamic theories are generally interested in interpreting behavior and this is important when trying to understand what makes people tick. In the scope of abstinence-based substance use treatment, it is a luxury and often comes down the road in one's recovery. To continue our sinking ship metaphor, people first have to get off the boat.

Years after the Titanic sank, theorists speculated about what went wrong, wrote books about it, and filmed movies.

CHAPTER 8

Cognitive Behavioral Theories

Cognitive Behavior Therapies. Cognitive behavioral therapies (CBT) are a collection of theories aimed at minimizing/eliminating negative, undesired behaviors and increasing positive ones (Corey, 2009; Pervin et al., 2005). CBT rejects psychodynamic theory that maladaptive behavior is the result of underlying issues and CBT does not emphasize some of the interpretative, self-focused and examining approaches of humanistic perspectives (Corey, 2009; Pervin et al., 2005). Instead, CBT focuses on current behavior and utilizes a scientific approach (Corey, 2009; Pervin et al., 2005). The behavior itself is considered to be the problem and it becomes the target. These approaches commonly believe that cognitive (thinking) processes affect behavior and that changing one's thinking can change one's behavior (Corey, 2009; Pervin et al., 2005).

Behavioral Therapy. There are two underlying principles that behavior therapies have in common – classical conditioning and operant conditioning (Corey, 2009; Pervin et al., 2005). Classical conditioning is the principle of learning based on Ivan Pavlov's work with gastric secretions with dogs (Corey, 2009). In the course of his studies, Pavlov placed food powder in the dogs' mouths and noticed the salivation. After many trials, he became aware that the dogs began to salivate even before the food was placed in the mouths; they saw the food dish, they knew the experimenter and so forth. He also rang a bell and the dogs would salivate at the sound of the bell. Stimuli that originally did not produce salivation could now produce salivation. This may not seem like a revelation, but it formed the basis for classical conditioning and has broad implications. The main principle at work here is that previously neutral stimuli can produce an elicited response based on association with stimuli that originally produces the response. In other words, if you have been stopped on the road for a traffic violation, the mere sight of a police car can now create apprehension.

There are three therapies based on classical conditioning: systematic desensitization, aversive conditioning, and assertiveness training (Corey, 2009; Pervin et al., 2005) Through systematic desensitization, the client learns to respond to previously anxiety- producing stimuli with a new, conditioned response of relaxation. The client is trained to relax. While in a relaxed state, the client is introduced to the anxiety-producing theme. If they become anxious, they are to return to a methodical relaxed state. The exercise is repeated until the client is able to remain relaxed while thinking about the anxiety-producing theme. This is typically accomplished in the therapy session.

Aversive therapy involves repeatedly combining an unconditioned stimulus that produces an undesirable response with an undesirable factor. Jail and/or probation is aversive therapy to the extreme. This eventually will lead to an avoidance of the unconditioned stimulus. In this case, the use of drugs/alcohol is the unconditioned stimulus when coupled with jail or the thought of it (the undesirable response) leads to avoiding drug/alcohol use.

Assertiveness training involves behavior rehearsal, modeling, and relaxation. The rehearsed response will replace an undesired maladaptive response in a given situation.

B. F. Skinner is considered the father of operant conditioning who believed that we get either positive or negative reinforcement or feedback from our social environment, which shapes our behavior (Corey, 2009; Pervin et al., 2005). Our behavior is either encouraged or discouraged by rewards and punishments.

Comment for the Reader: There are numerous applications of CBT methods and techniques used in drug and alcohol counseling. Psycho-education groups employ CBT. Most programs utilize CBT skills; sometimes they are more like classes that teach a variety of skills aimed at providing new coping strategies for common triggers to use drugs/alcohol. Triggers include, but are not limited to: work, money, boredom, relationships, anger, friends and family, cravings, mental illness, loneliness, hunger, tiredness, and so forth. These coping strategies are not unlike methods found in Positive Psychology, which involves clients engaging in behaviors that enhance happiness.

Another example involves the use of contingency contracts, which may be written with clients. These contracts spell out given consequences and rewards for given behavior. It exemplifies operant behavior. Interestingly, members at 12-Step groups can receive tokens or key chains for lengths of sobriety/abstinence. It is a traditional experience at many meetings. What it does is set up an environment that rewards appropriate, desirable behavior, which is periodically reinforced. I know, though, no one thinks of AA as behavioral therapy!

Rational Emotive Therapy. Albert Ellis is the founder of RET which is sometimes considered to be in the humanistic school of psychology, but because it involves cognitive processes, it is being presented with the CBT theories. RET looks at a set of circumstances and creates a formula where "A" is the environmental event that the individual is presented with; "B" is the thought they have in response to "A," and "C" is the emotional behavior they have in response to "B" (Corey, 2009; Ellis, 2005). The theory is that our behavior is based on our thinking – not an external event. The counselor tries to help the client alter irrational ideas they have in response to events (Corey, 2009;

(also enjoy the positive effects of rational thinking.)

Ellis, 2005). Ellis believed that people made irrational or unrealistic demands on themselves and others as a result of judging, and rating themselves and others, as well as making over-generalizations about people, behavior, and life situations (Corey, 2009; Ellis, 2005). For example, if a child is laughed at for crying in school, they might learn it is best not to cry because crying is wrong and bad. They then feel poorly about themselves any time they want to cry. The counselor's goal is to replace the client's irrational and faulty beliefs with healthy ones.

> *Comment for the Reader:* The most common usage of RET is seen in Rational Recovery (RR) Groups, an alternative to AA. RR does not involve the use of a 'Higher Power' and utilizes the "ABC" theory of behavior, cognitive processes, and method for change.

CHAPTER 9

HUMANISTIC THEORY

In order to get off that sinking boat quickly there are many "here and now" theories framed as phenomenological/humanistic approaches which focus on changing one's behavior. They assist people in identifying their thoughts and feelings, and developing solutions to problems.

Existential Therapy. This is an interesting perspective which falls into the phenomenological/humanistic/experiential view of therapy (as opposed to psychodynamic or behavioral perspectives). R. May (1969) indicates it has to do with finding meaning in life; it emphasizes human experiences. Existential therapy focuses on the individual's exploration for values in their life, personal freedom, self-fulfillment, and purpose in what would otherwise be a meaningless, uncaring, and lonely world (Corey, 2009). Rollo May, founder of existential therapy, identifies anxiety as the conflicts that arise in the pursuit of that self-actualization. Corey, 2009, explains that existential anxiety is that which arises when exercising choices and decisions in a realm of uncertainty. It becomes very philosophical. Existential therapy avoids the use of any methods and techniques, and emphasizes the relationship between counselor and client as partners in an attempt to establish the client's identity in the world (Corey, 2009). While the counselor does not represent an authority, or attempt to direct the client, he does point out pros and cons, and alternatives of the client's thoughts, actions, and decisions. The counselor may use self-disclosure and model authentic living.

> *Comment for the Reader:* Existential therapy is one of the few therapies that encourage the counselor's self-disclosure. From this perspective, it hints of an AA sponsor type of relationship in that the counselor has partnered with the client in an effort for the client to make order of his life and the sponsor, of course, serves as a model for the client. Existential approach also fits right in with the hopeless client who is experiencing a bottom and searching for a way to survive, recover, and find a way of life that is feasible, workable, sustaining, and fulfilling. Once again we see another explanation for anxiety, but more importantly it suggests the major role that anxiety plays in drug/alcohol usage and in particular, in its relationship to reaching personal goals. The search for meaning and purpose hits home for the client who is experiencing crisis after crisis and/or a lot of drama in their lives.

Gestalt Therapy. Gestalt is a concept that basically means the whole is greater than the sum of its parts. A goal of gestalt therapy is to help the client reach maturity through self-responsibility and integration (Perls et al., 1951; Corey, 2009). Integration means gaining awareness in order to unify the self into maturity for self-actualization in life (Perls et al., 1951; Corey, 2009). In other words, it aims to assist people to grow and enhance their potential. The emphasis is on the direct experience and doing, as opposed to talking about feelings. The client focuses on what and how, but not why (Perls et al., 1951; Corey, 2009). It is about the process not about technique. The process is about what is happening here and now (Perls et al., 1951; Corey, 2009). By becoming aware of choices, people assume responsibility and develop meaning in their lives. People seek closure for unfinished business (Perls et al., 1951; Corey, 2009). Unfinished business represents unexpressed anger, sadness, disappointment, guilt, grief, and so forth. These feelings linger and affect present behavior, and interfere with relationships and reaching one's potential and highest quality of life (Perls et al., 1951; Corey, 2009). Unfinished business can torment an individual and affect their present behavior. People may often avoid unresolved issues rather than make necessary changes. People reach impasses and get stuck in current behavior due to layers of blockage. Clients are asked to begin statements with "I" in order to assume responsibility for their actions (Perls et al., 1951; Corey, 2009).

Comment for the Reader: Gestalt Therapy offers several useful concepts for drug/alcohol counseling. The first is the notion of self-responsibility. The addict/alcoholic may not be responsible for being addicted/alcoholic, but once they are, they are responsible/accountable for treatment for it. Some theories hold that the addict/alcoholic is born that way (see addiction theory in Unit 1); that may be so, but upon coming to terms with one's addiction comes a responsibility to follow a protocol. The client uses "I" statements, which can assist breaking through denial of a problem. Focusing on a 'what' and 'how' approach in the 'here' and 'now' is also beneficial. The 'what' and 'how' spells out what to do for recovery and how to do it. It presents the client with choices of how to handle situations. Working in the present reiterates our 'get off the boat' analogy. Now, while unfinished business must be dealt with, one proceeds with how it affects the client in the present; the feelings and behaviors that are occurring presently as a result of unresolved issues.

Reality Therapy. William Glasser is the founder of Reality Therapy. He bases it on the need and struggle for one's identity (Glasser, 1990). Identity is composed of two related concepts; the need to be loved and the need to feel worthwhile (Glasser, 1990). Reality therapy makes a distinction between a success identity and a failure identity (Glasser, 1990). In other words, how we perceive ourselves can determine how we reach goals. Glasser views it to be the responsibility of the individual to fulfill their needs and sees problems as a result of irresponsibility and a failure identity. The goal of therapy thus is to become responsible to fill one's needs and adopt a success identity (Glasser, 1990). Reality therapy does not look at dysfunction as a mental illness and focuses on present behaviors, encourages a realistic communication level between counselor and client, and emphasizes the client's ability to figure out what is right or wrong in their life (Glasser, 1990). Reality therapy then helps to teach the client how to go about meeting their needs (Glasser, 1990).

Comment for the Reader: What I like about reality therapy in terms of substance abuse counseling is the notion of failure/ success identities. It further exemplifies the part that low self-esteem plays in continuing substance use. Reality therapy also supports CBT type skill and strategy building for the client to meet their needs.

Narrative Therapy. Narrative therapy is an emerging treatment approach from Martin Payne. Narrative therapy is a relatively simple theory that has powerful implications for the client. Basically, it suggests that how we perceive our lives has a big impact on how we shape our lives accordingly (Payne, 2006). In other words, if a client's story is wrought with failure, inadequacies, hopeless situations, victimizations, and so forth, this can manifest itself in the client's life. It works like a self-fulfilled prophecy. In other words, that which a client perceives in their lives becomes what presents itself in their lives. In narrative therapy, the client is encouraged to share their story (Payne, 2006). The counselor then assists the client in reshaping their story (Payne, 2006). Clients may misrepresent events in their lives or have misunderstandings of those events and this is believed to be unhealthy. The counselor helps the client 'reauthor' their story in order to pave the way for positive change (Payne, 2006). The counselor listens to the client's story and looks for prevailing influences that impact on the client's life that might explain events (Payne, 2006).

Comment for the Reader. Our story is a powerful thing. We can see this with the role that the story has in 12 Step programs. The program encourages its members to take a "fearless and moral inventory" of their lives (the 4th step). This is most certainly based on the members' perceptions of their lives or their stories, if you will. The inventory is an account of a member's life. In the 5th step, the member shares this inventory with another person. A sponsor, or clergyman, or counselor may help the member to see patterns of behavior and even adopt new ways of looking at their lives which pave the way for steps six thru nine (see the 12-step section). Also, at speaker meetings, members share their stories. This is intended to provide identification and inspiration for the group. Usually the speaker has a period of sobriety under their belt. The early recovery speaker's story is apt to be wrought with devastation, whereas the seasoned member in recovery has been around long enough to reframe their story from a new perspective. The story, as recovering 12-step members are aware, is a powerful theme in recovery and meetings. In discussion meetings, members often share parts of their story. It is important to remember, we all have a story and how we tell it impacts greatly on how we perceive our lives.

Client-Centered Therapy. Client-centered therapy is also known as person-centered therapy (PCT). It has become widely accepted for use not only in substance use/dual diagnosis treatment, but also in many other aspects of the health care field. It has become not only a therapy method and technique, but also an approach to helping people in general, and has become the paradigm (an accepted perspective) of this era in health care. Therefore, we will talk about PCT in greater detail and devote more time to it.

Historical Development. Person-centered therapy was fostered and developed by Carl Rogers (1902-1987) in the 1940s and 1950s (Kirshenbaum, 2004). Parlier, Neubaum, and Simkins (2002) describe the times. This was a patriarchal time as the popular TV show 'Father Knows Best' portrayed, a family America aspired to be – happy and dressing for dinner together. The Cold War began to loom over us with the threat of nuclear war with the Soviets. Bomb shelters were built and we practiced crawling under our desks in school. There was the Sputnik threat – a Soviet satellite supposedly to spy on us. Plessy and Ferguson explain why African Americans can no longer be treated under the "separate, but equal" rule. It forecast the future of civil rights and assured Americans that full integration was inevitable. Rosa Parks refused to go to the back of the bus. Swanson TV dinners were the rave. Girls took 'home economics' in school. We waged war in Korea and Jackie Robinson waged a different kind of war on the baseball field as our first African American professional baseball player. Americans began a love affair with their automobiles.

Kirshenbaum (2004) reports on Rogers' life. Rogers was born outside of Chicago; his parents were conservative, Protestant, Midwesterners. He had a strong religious upbringing. As a teen, his family purchased a farm in Illinois and Rogers first decided to be a farmer. At the University of Wisconsin, he experienced a call to religious work and switched his major from agriculture to history in order to prepare for the ministry. He also took psychology courses and progressive education, and was influenced by John Dewey's education philosophy. Dewey believed that students should be involved in real-life tasks and challenges. Rogers pursued a doctorate in clinical psychology. He encountered Freudian thought, lectures by Adler, Rorschach testing, and other psychoanalytic and psychiatric approaches. While working on his dissertation, Rogers lived in Rochester, NY, and was influenced by Jessie Taft, a student of Otto Rank. Their focus shifted from a past reference to 'relationship therapy' and looked at a patient's insight and self-acceptance within the therapeutic relationship.

Kirshenbaum (2004) continues. Rogers taught at Ohio State University where he popularized the term "client" as opposed to "patient." He emphasized that people should not be deemed dependent on their doctor, but as a responsible individual and that those in psychological distress were not necessarily 'sick.' His hypothesis was that the client had the capacity within himself to understand his difficulties and strive toward his potential (self-actualizing) in such a way to achieve internal comfort (Ford & Mass, 1989). Rogers developed a "non-directive method" and avoided asking questions, interpretation, suggestions, advice, or other directive techniques. He relied on a process of listening to the client, unconditional regard for the client, and reflecting back the client's feelings. This blurred the boundaries between counseling and psychotherapy; counseling applied to mild problems of adjustment and psychotherapy to more deep-seated problems. Rogers was suggesting that all problems could be applied to a continuum of adjustment. He was the first person to publish cases of psychotherapy. This earned his innovative approach a seat in theoretical orientations.

The evolution of PCT can be divided into four phases (Pervin, Cervone, & Oliver, 2005; Corey, 2009).

1) 1940-1950: Nondirective psychotherapy. This approach emphasized that the counselor remained somewhat passive and did not intervene in the client's decision-making. Through this environment, clients could develop insight into themselves and their life situations.
2) 1950-1957: Reflective psychotherapy. During this period the counselor reflected the clients' feelings back to them and remained non-threatening or challenging in the relationship. Through this reflective therapy, the client moves closer from their self-concept to their ideal self and their actualizing potential.
3) 1957-1970: Experiential therapy. This approach included the counselor's expression of basic ideas. The counselor's role was to emphasize his responsiveness to the clients' feelings. This period introduced the counselor's attitude of congruence, positive regard, acceptance, and empathic understanding as prerequisites of effective therapy. The counselor now includes his feelings and opinions as well as reflecting the clients' feelings.
4) 1970s forward. The new emphasis included greater involvement on the part of the therapist as a person by sharing their thoughts, feelings, and values and willing to use them in the therapeutic process. This allows for a greater range and flexibility of counselor behavior, which in earlier periods was undesirable. Previously, the counselor was discouraged from setting goals, giving advice, and interpreting behavior. Now there is more of an eclectic spirit in using a wider variety of methods. The aim, however, is still to create an atmosphere in which the client feels fully accepted and can grow in (Pervin, Cervone, & Oliver, 2005).

Major Assumptions. Rogers also recognized that it was the therapeutic relationship that fosters growth in the client and that 3 conditions existed (Cheston, 2000; Pervin et al., 2005; Corey, 2009). 1) Unconditional positive regard. 2) Empathy. 3) Genuineness and authenticity. Rogers believed clients do not need judgment, interpretation, advice, or direction, but supportive counselors to help them achieve their own insights and direction. Rogers wrote many books, among which was "On Becoming a Person: A Therapist's View." This became associated with what Maslow termed as a third force in psychology, implying psychoanalysis, behaviorism, and now "humanistic psychology" (Ziegler, 2002).

The historical perspectives merge into three major tenets of client-centered therapy (Corey, 2009; Pervin et al., 2005; Rogers, 1989; Rogers, 1988). The counselor must possess an unconditional positive regard for the client and sincerely care about them. Parents are usually the first source of unconditional and conditional regard. As an adult, the clients become their own source for positive regard. The counselor remains non-judgmental and accepting of the client. The counselor may not be pleased with all the client's actions, but he remains accepting of the client and non-judgmental. Judgments are considered conditions of worth both positive and negative.

The second tenet is for the counselor to provide the client with empathic understanding. The counselor must listen and reflect back to the client an understanding of how the client feels.

Lastly, the counselor must be genuine and honest with the client in order to generate trust between themselves and the client. Early client-centered therapy was meant to be non-directive so that the counselor was not an authority figure and avoided advice giving, interpretation, and diagnosing. Rogers felt that the client was their own expert of their life. As client-centered therapy evolved, there was a certain shift from the counselor merely reflecting back the client's feeling to including the therapist's own immediate feelings, thoughts, opinions, and so forth, which created a greater range and flexibility for the counselor depending upon the needs of the client.

Humanism gave emphasis to the client's experience and frame of reference as opposed to evaluating and diagnosing. It focused on not just problem-solving, but self-actualizing. Humanism centered on choice, will, freedom, values, feelings, and goals. (Corey, 2009).

A consistent theme underlies Rogers' theories; a deep faith in the human tendency to develop in a positive and constructive way if a climate of respect and trust exists between client and counselor. (Pervin, Cervone, & Oliver, 2005; Corey, 2009; Rogers, 1988; Rogers, 1989). He criticized the Freudian preoccupation with the sick and crippled side of human nature. He did not believe therapist should be superior or in an 'expert' position. The positive view of human nature has significant implications for counseling. (Pervin, Cervone, & Oliver, 2005). Because the client has the inherent ability for wellness, the therapist places the primary responsibility on the client (Rogers, 1988; Rogers, 1989). This is a highly axiological approach (a theoretical perspective that is founded in value; in this case, PCT places great significance on the client's responsibility to oneself). Therapy is rooted in the client's capacity for awareness and the ability to make decisions. Seeing people in this light, means the counselor can focus on constructive directions and how the client can successfully deal with obstacles blocking their growth (i.e., substance abuse).

Stategies. The therapeutic aims of PCT differ from traditional approaches. PCT works toward a greater degree of independence for the client (Pervin, Cervone, & Oliver, 2005). The focus is on the person not the presenting problem (Corey, 2009). The strategy is not merely for the client to solve their problems, but to assist in the growing process. The counselor wants to establish a climate conducive toward helping the client become a fully functioning person (Corey, 2009). Rogers describe the actualizing person as open to experience, developing a trust in themselves, developing an internal sense of evaluation, and possessing a willingness to grow (Pervin, Cervone, & Oliver, 2005; Rogers, 1988).

Rogers believed that people possessed an innate ability to be all they can be, to reach their potential, and "self-actualize" (Corey, 2009; Pervin et al., 2005; Rogers, 1989; Rogers, 1988). Rogers (1989, 1988) explains his ideas in detail. He theorized that people have a set of perceptions of themselves in relation to the world around them. When a person experiences conditions for their worthiness, this is called incongruence. Conditions of worthiness are when an individual feels they are not worthy unless they__________. (Fill in the blank.) These conditions usually come from messages received from parents during childhood. Incongruence creates anxiety. People often distort their perceptions and use denial as a result. This may help to alleviate some anxiety, but does help them realized their potential. Client-centered therapy operates on the premise that if the counselor sets the right climate, the client can alleviate anxiety, achieve congruence, and come closer to meeting their goals. Rogers believed that real positive personality change can only occur within a relationship and self-intellectualizing is not sufficient. He believed that if the right climate occurs, the client possesses the capacity for growth and change.

Being open to experience means seeing reality without distorting it to fit into preconceived ideas about themselves. It means that one's ideas are not rigid and that the individual can grow and tolerate ambiguity. One goal of therapy is for the client to develop a sense of trust in themselves (Pervin, Cervone, & Oliver, 2005). Clients coming into treatment are not likely to trust themselves or their decisions very much. Related to self-trust is developing a sense of being one's own counsel (Rogers, 1989). It means learning to look to oneself for the answers to one's problems. The client learns to decide his own standards of behavior and looks to himself to make decisions and choices to live by.

Continuing to grow means accepting the idea that life is a process; we are always becoming and actualizing. We do not become 'actualized' (Pervin, Cervone, & Oliver, 2005). We are not like a pie we put in the oven and take out when it is baked. Clients often look for a recipe for being happy and successful – an end product. Instead, the client learns to realize that life is a process. These characteristics provide a framework therapy. The counselor does not choose specific goals for the client. The client develops his own.

The role of the PCT counselor is more a way of being than a technique (Rogers, 1988; Rogers, 1989). Their purpose is to establish a climate within which the client can grow (Corey, 2009). The client must feel the freedom to explore areas of their life. If they are not defensive, they will be much more open to different possibilities (Pervin et al., 2005). Most importantly, the counselor must be willing to be real in their relationship with the client. It is through the counselor's ability to be genuine, caring, respectful, accepting, and understanding that the client feels comfortable enough to grow and move to a higher level of functioning (Pervin, Cervone, & Oliver, 2005).

In practice. In the early 1980s, the epistemological paradigm (the basis for the theory of knowledge in the field) was a problem-focused, deficit/needs-based approach. It involved an expert-based therapy and behavioral-oriented treatment. Alcoholics Anonymous (AA) was heavily prescribed as the only thing out there to promote continued sobriety. In the mid 1990s, we began to see a shift toward client-centered treatment and the client was brought into the treatment planning and goal-setting process. Harm reduction strategies have tacitly been embraced. This emanates from the National Institute of Mental Health (NIMH) and the Substance Abuse and Mental Health Services Administration (SAMHSA) and has filtered its way down to state and community level. Government-funded agencies have adopted a philosophy of treatment that encompasses various ideologies and techniques in substance abuse and mental health treatment. They include Recovery Core Values, Integrated Dual Diagnosis Treatment (IDDT), Motivational Interviewing, Stages of Change, and Harm Reduction Theories. These concepts are intertwined, but identifiable. They all have PCT as a grounding foundation.

Recovery Core Values are ethical principles applied to mental illness and substance abuse. There are three basic premises. All persons in recovery are individuals with individual needs and perspectives about their health and behavior. People in recovery with mental illness, substance abuse, or both, share some similarities. Managing their lives will require different venues at times. All individuals have an equal opportunity to attain treatment and recovery (Andres-Hyman, 2004).

Those in recovery must have the opportunity to participate in their treatment planning. Every effort is made to provide services that are culturally diverse. Service providers will respect the individual's choice in treatment direction (Andres-Hyman, 2004).

Prochaski, DiClemente, and Norcross (1992) developed the stages of change. Motivational Interviewing (Scherling, 2004) began to be used to gently move people through stages of change (see Chapter 16). Around 2000, harm-reduction theories (MacMaster, 2004) (see Chapter 5), were reintroduced and fit in nicely with a client-centered approach. AA is still highly recommended. but it is proposed in conjunction with other CBT/solutions-focused strategies. This went along with strengths-based techniques and an Integrated Dual Diagnosis Treatment (IDDT) approach (Andres-Hyman, 2004). Integrated Dual Diagnosis Treatment (IDDT) is basically a combination of these Recovery Core Values and Motivational Interviewing (MI).

To recap these ideologies, autonomy and self-determination (the first guiding principle of the American Counseling Association ACA code of ethics) are the hallmark of Recovery Core Values, Stages of Change, and Motivational Interviewing – perhaps, to a fault when implementing substance abuse treatment. At times, drug and alcohol treatment require a much stronger directive, sometimes confrontational, role on behalf of the counselor.

A vulnerability of PCT is the tendency of some counselors to give support to clients without challenging them. Out of a misunderstanding of the basic concepts, some counselors have limited the range of their repertoire to styles of reflection and empathic listening. As a result, the client may not receive much needed direction and guidance.

The heart of the matter, though, is that some substance abuse counselors, do not always recommend abstinence and attendance at Alcoholics Anonymous, an abstinence- based program, as treatment objectives. This writer conducted informal interviews with six healthcare providers at a former agency. The parameters herein do not permit an in-depth review of those interviews. However, results indicated that most did not believe that the clients (in this case, profound, severe, and chronically mentally ill) were capable of remaining abstinent and opted to use a harm-reduction approach. This is an injustice to these clients. Many can and do adopt an abstinent lifestyle, but they may need to be challenged to do so. The Stages of Change and Motivational Interviewing are methods that are devised to do so.

> *Comment for the Reader:* In summation, there has been a paradigm (theoretical approach) shift in substance abuse counseling from a needs-based approach to a strengths-based approach. In other words, instead of focusing on the clients' 'deficits,' the counselor instead focuses on the clients' 'strengths.' Psychodynamic theories tended to look at the clients' deficiencies; client-centered approach is a method to enhance the clients' positive factors. Also, client-centered therapy takes on a more collaborative approach; the therapist takes a less authoritative role and the client ideally leads in the

choice of direction and treatment. One of the most important things we take from client-centered therapy is this idea of a strong therapeutic alliance. This refers to the relationship the counselor has with the client. The counselor needs to be unconditionally accepting, warm, genuine, and empathic. This creates the nurturing environment the clients need to find their own solutions. The humanistic perspective broke from the traditional therapist role as the expert and authority in early doctor-patient roles. Certainly, there are times when the counselor needs to be action and direction oriented. The client may need to be told the boat is sinking and provided with ways to get off and to find a safe way to shore and shelter. This is discussed in the cognitive-behavioral section. But the point here is that more than one approach is necessary when dealing with the substance use client and the counselor must be comfortable shifting gear, depending on the needs of the client. Client-centered therapy is today's method of choice, but counselors who rely on early versions of this approach and mostly use empathic listening, allowing the client to solely navigate may be too passive. Addiction/alcoholism is a disease of denial and the seriousness of the situation and consequences often needs to be driven home because the client can't see it. Often, this can be done in a gentle and kind way, as we will see with motivational interviewing. The days of shaving addicts' heads and scrubbing latrines are long gone. However, there are times, as indicated, when things need to be pointed out to the client in no uncertain terms.

CHAPTER 10

The Paradigm Shift

There has been a paradigm (a model of underlying beliefs) shift from needs-based therapy to a strengths-based perspectives, person-centered therapy that we will talk about a lot. Both mental health and substance abuse practitioners have historically viewed clients based on their needs or deficits, which was founded in traditional psychodynamic psychology. As the prevailing school of thought has shifted to a humanistic, existential direction, there has been an increased effort to base treatment on a clients' strengths which forms the basis of integrated dual diagnosis treatment (IDDT). The National Substance Abuse and Mental Health Administration's (SAMHSA) proposed model of recovery and recovery-oriented services includes several basic recovery premises.

Andres-Hyman (2004) discuss these principles. First, all clients are individual and have specific needs, objectives, attitudes, behaviors, and expectations for recovery. Clients, whether being treated for mental health issues, substance abuse, or both, have things in common; however, the directions and pursuits that people choose may be different. Clients are encouraged to actively participate in their treatment and recovery process. Treatment must be approached holistically. Clients must be able to collaborate in every determining phase of their treatment plan. Nomenclature will reflect individualized recovery-based language; i.e., "Recovery Plans" shall replace "Treatment Plans." This strengths-based approach shall be used and promoted. There should not be any "wrong doors" when entering treatment service. A client's choice must be respected in all matters. Programming must be flexible to incorporate individual recovery plans.

Andres-Hyman (2004) continue discussing core values. IDDT has determined that there are several Recovery Dimensions. They include understanding how behaviors effect recovery; hope, confidence and commitment; understanding and accepting oneself; relationships with family, friends, and supportive of others; maintaining recovery; supports in the community to enhance recovery; promoting recovery; and becoming an empowered citizen.

While the objectives of these Recovery Core Values are clear about dealing with the client as an individual, in a strengths-based fashion, and in a collaborative manner, we do not turn the client away who says, "I don't want to stop using drugs" because they don't agree with OUR goal for them to be abstinent. It is vital that we meet clients where they are without confrontation, condescension, judgment, or disapproval, because we run the risk of losing them altogether. Better that we can keep them in treatment to engage with them for another day.

But, "what happened to helping someone be drug-free?" you say. We still do but we go about it differently. The upcoming section (Chapter 15) regarding Motivational Interviewing (MI) will explain in greater detail, but basically MI is a kinder, gentler way of instilling hope for a better life than the confrontational Daytop (an acronym for "Drug Addicts Yielding to Persuasion," an early prominent trend-setting treatment facility started in NY in 1963) days of shaving heads and cleaning latrines.

So, all of that is to say that we collaborate with the client in setting up an individualized treatment plan. We meet them where they are. That "paradigm shift" means that our role has changed; we are not the "expert" or the "director" – the client is in the driver's seat. Remember that Rogers' person-centered therapy is based on the belief that the clients have within themselves the capacity and the ability to solve their own problems, given the right environment. Our job is, through our authenticity, genuineness, warmth, acceptance, and 'unconditional regard' for the client, to create the type of supportive atmosphere where the client can grow, change, and reach their potential.

CONCLUSION

Various counseling approaches have been presented in this unit. Are one or more theories of particular interest to you? It is my hope that many of your own ideas are finding a theoretical home that you are comfortable with and that as you read you have said to yourself . . . "well, I knew that . . ." or "of course, that just makes sense. . . ."

In the next unit, we take a closer look at the role Alcoholics Anonymous has played in treatment of drug addiction as well as the relationship between conventional counseling and AA. They are not different and separate, but truly complement each other.

UNIT 2 Highlights

CH 7/Psychodynamic Theory

- Freud, Adler, Jung/major theorists
- Interpretative (vs. problem solving)
- Conflict centered in the past (vs. here and now)
- Transference is emotions and attitudes client puts onto counselor from parental or other powerful relationships/ Counter transference is counselor's conflict elicited from client

CH 8/Cognitive/Behavioral Theories

- Minimizes/eliminates negative undesired behavior/increases positive desired behavior
- Pavlov/Classical Conditioning/neutral stimulus can produce elicited response by association to original stimulus
- Systematic desensitization/aversion therapy/assertiveness training
- Skinner/Operant Conditioning/positive and negative reinforcement
- Rational Emotive Therapy/event 'A' elicits response 'B' elicits action 'C'

CH 9/Humanistic Theory

- "Here and now"
- Changing behavior by identifying thoughts and feelings, and developing solutions to problems
- Existential Theory/finding meaning in life
- GestaltTheory/key concepts/self-responsibility/integration/ unfinished business

- Reality Theory/self-responsibility to fill one's need to be loved and feel worthwhile/failure-success identity shapes life
- Narrative Theory/how we perceive our life has large implications
- Person-centered therapy/Carl Rogers
- PCT key concepts/therapeutic alliance/unconditional positive regard/empathy/genuineness and authenticity/deep faith in client's ability to solve their own problems in the right climate/actualizing/the basis for new paradigm in integrated dual diagnosis treatment
- The new paradigm represents a shift from a needs-based perspective to a strengths-based one, emphasizing the client's role in their treatment

STUDY GUIDE

1) Which counseling theory resonates with you?
2) What is it about you, your personality, your history, and so forth that leads you to connect with your theory of choice?
3) What is the shift of paradigm? Why do you think it is important?

References

Andres-Hyman, R. (2004, December). *Recovery Core Values.* Handout Presented at Connecticut Department of Mental Health and Addiction Services Education and Training, Hartford, CT.

Booth, K.; Kenrick, M.; & Woods, S. (1997). Nursing knowledge, theory, and method revisited. *Journal of Advanced Nursing*, 26(4), 804-811.

Cheston, S.E. (2004). A new paradigm for teaching counseling theory and practice. Counselor Education and Supervision, 39(4), 254-270.

Clark, A.M. (1998). The qualitative-quantitative debate: moving from positivism and confrontation to post-positivism and reconciliation. *Journal of Advanced Nursing,* 27(6),1242-1249.

Corey, G. (2009). *Theory and practice of counseling and psychotherapy* (8th ed.). Belmont, CA: Brooks/Cole.

Cramer, D. & Takens, R.J. (1992). Therapeutic relationship and progress in the first six sessions of individual psychotherapy: A panel analysis. *Counseling Psychology Quarterly,* 5(1), 25-36.

CT Certification Board (n.d.). Retrieved from http://www.ctcertboard.org/ on February 2, 2008.

Ellis, A. (2005). *Rational emotive behavior therapy.* Atascadero, CA: Impact Publishers.

Ford, G.J. & Mass, S. (1989). On actualizing person-centered theory: A critique of textbook treatments of Rogers' motivational constructs. *Teaching of Psychology,* 16(1), 30-31.

Glasser, W. (1990) *Reality therapy: A new approach to psychiatry.* NY: Harper Row, Publishers.

Kirshenbaum, H. (2004). Carl Rogers' life and work: An assessment on the 100th anniversary of his birth. *Journal of Counseling and Development,* 82(1), 166-125.

LaChance, A. (2005). *Psychology and spirituality: How to help your clients and heal the human psyche.* Handout at presentation of Cross Country Education. Hartford, CT.

MacMaster, S.A. (2004). Harm reduction: a new perspective on substance abuse services [Electronic Version] *Social Work,* 49(3), 356-364.

May, R. (1969). *Existential psychology.* NY: Random House.

Onweugbuzie, A.J. (2002). Why can't we all get along? Toward a framework for unifying research paradigms. Education, 122(3), 518-531.

Parlier, S.; Neubaum, J.; Simkins, J. (2002). Behind the picket fence: National history project, Illinois State University retrieved from http://www.history.ilstu.edu/nhp/civilization/Site/welcome.html on January 19, 2008.

Patterson, T.G. (2006). Development of a self-report measure of unconditional positive self-regard. Psychology and Psychotherapy: Theory, Research, and Practice, 79(4), 557-570.

Payne, M. (2006). *Narrative therapy.* Thousand Oaks, CA: Sage Publications.

Pervin, L.; Cervone, D.; & Oliver, J. (2005). *Theories of personality.* Hoboken, NJ: John Wiley & Sons, Inc.

Prochaska, J.O.; Diclemente, C.C.; Norcross, J.C. (1992). In search of how people change: applications to addictive behaviors [Electronic Version] *American Psychologist,* 47(9), 1102-1114.

Rogers, C. (1989). *Client-centered therapy.* London: Constable & Robinson, Ltd.

Rogers, C. (1988). *On becoming a person.* NY: Houghton Mifflin Co.

Scherling, D.H. (2004, October). *Hopeful Conversations: Inspiring Recovery Through Motivational Interviewing.* Handout Presented at Connecticut Department of Mental Health and Addiction Services Education and Training, Middletown, CT.

Ziegler, D.J. (2002). Freud, Rogers, and Ellis: A comparative theoretical analysis. *Journal of Rational-Emotive and Cognitive-Behavioral Therapy*, 20(2), 75-91.

UNIT 3/12-Step Theory

Introduction

Alcoholics Anonymous has laid the foundation for the treatment of alcoholism and other drug addictions; it has been one of the first and only approaches for many years. It is important to understand the role AA has played in the field today. In recent years, it has received much criticism, some of which is founded on misconceptions and a misunderstanding of AA philosophy. One valid point, however, is that AA is not for everyone and that there can be more than one approach to recovery.

CHAPTER 11

AA Philosophy in Treatment Programs

The 12 Steps of Alcoholics Anonymous are as follows:

1. We admitted we were powerless over alcohol – that our lives had become unmanageable.
2. Came to believe that a Power greater than ourselves could restore us to sanity.
3. Made a decision to turn our will and our lives over to the care of God *as we understood Him.*
4. Made a searching and fearless moral inventory of ourselves.
5. Admitted to God, to ourselves, and to another human being the exact nature of our wrongs.
6. Were entirely ready to have God remove all these defects of character.
7. Humbly asked Him to remove our shortcomings.
8. Made a list of all persons we had harmed, and became willing to make amends to them all.

9. Made direct amends to such people wherever possible, except when to do so would injure them or others.
10. Continued to take personal inventory and when we were wrong promptly admitted it.
11. Sought through prayer and meditation to improve our conscious contact with God, *as we understood Him,* praying only for knowledge of His will for us and the power to carry that out.
12. Having had a spiritual awakening as the result of these Steps, we tried to carry this message to alcoholics, and to practice these principles in all our affairs.

While it is certainly understood by treatment providers today, that AA and its variant 12-Step Programs (OA, CA, GA, and so forth) are not the only thing going in terms of recovery, the 12-Step process remains strong. There are an estimated 2 million members of AA alone worldwide, 1million estimated in the United States, and over 100,000 groups worldwide.

There are both adversarial and complementary forces at play between AA and traditional mental health treatments that are worth taking a look at. We are in an age of a dual diagnosis paradigm, and while most treatment facilities used to be based in AA philosophy, this has changed greatly since the 1990s.

AA has suffered from much criticism. In the past, in early recovery treatment centers, spirituality was interwoven with Alcoholics Anonymous, as facilities were AA oriented. Spirituality became controversial. Questions of the AA message lowering an individual's self-esteem due to their "powerlessness" as stated in Step 1, and the program's religiosity were leveled due to the inclusion of the expressive concepts of "God" and "a Power greater than ourselves."

As stated in early substance abuse treatment, Alcoholics Anonymous (AA) was the preferred (and virtually only) approach available. The words "God" and "Higher Power" are used freely throughout the literature, and while strong proponents of AA will expound on the distinction that AA is a spiritual program and not a religious program, many individuals are turned off.

Huguelet and Koenig (2009) distinguish between spirituality and religiosity in a way that provides a distinction between the two concepts. Accordingly, religion is considered to indicate "specific behavioral, social, doctrinal, and denominational characteristics" (p. 1). It includes the notion of a transcendent in a ritualistic and formalized manner. Spirituality is concerned with "ultimate questions of life's meaning" (p. 1) in a subjective way. The term spirituality eludes specific operational definitions. It is likely to differ when individuals speak of the spiritual, though it is generally referring to the non-material. It may or may not include religion. It often, however, may fall into four areas: a person's relationship with God; the deepest level from which a human being operates; the philosophical context of a person's life, including values, rules, attitudes and views; the same as religion (Ramson et al., 2005).

Critics suggest that the steps of AA lead the individual into esteem deterioration instead of proliferation by using concepts such as powerlessness and unmanageable, and the promotion of the use of a Higher Power as the only way out. There has been a certain trend away from AA and toward cognitive behavioral techniques because they are considered to be all-inclusive. AA is supported as ONE method of recovery, not the ONLY method of recovery. Spirituality is supported as one of many CBT methods to be employed. Any in-depth spirituality exploration is often not addressed due to its controversial nature, or referred out to faith-based providers.

In order to understand the conflict, controversy, and provocative nature of promoting spirituality in treatment programs, it is necessary to look at criticisms of Alcoholics Anonymous in treatment programs.

The main problem is that there is not a lot of empirical evidence supporting the efficacy of AA (Mackenzie, Alisdair, & Allen, 2003). This is despite the fact that AA and other 12 step programs based on it, remain the most popular treatment for alcohol and other drug abuse. This is demonstrated by the fact that on any given week, there may be thousands of AA meetings attended all over the world. There are seven major criticisms leveled against AA. From an AA insider's perspective, they are wrought with misconception.

First, by acknowledging "powerlessness over my addiction," AA takes power away from those who are already disenfranchised. The first step of AA states "We admitted we were powerless over alcohol and that our lives became unmanageable. It is also a major stumbling block for professionals and newcomers alike (Davis, Golie, & Jansen, 1998). In Western society, self-reliance is considered a powerful virtue. Accepting limitations, for many, goes against the "pull yourself up by the bootstraps" philosophy. Powerlessness implies defeat and on first impressions, one is not aware of AA's subtleties and metaphors. AA philosophies require information and learning before determining meaning and interpretation (Davis, Golie, & Jansen, 1998). "Powerlessness" in this case is like a Buddhist puzzle; i.e., one must lose their life in order to gain it; giving in is actually a form of control. A popular AA slogan is "Surrender to win!" Step 1 suggests a look at the hard fact of being out of control with drinking and/or other drugs. It invites people to survey their world and see that controlled usage doesn't work, hasn't worked, and won't work. The purpose is to convince the addict/alcoholic that change is necessary and that this is the first step in that change (Davis, Golie, & Jansen, 1998; Riordan & Walsh).

The second and third steps do deal with the notion of a Higher Power and this is the next area of criticism. The third step mentions "God" and critics connect this with a "suspiciously white, male, dominant-culture Christian God" (Davis, Rae, & Jansen, 1998, p. 173). Also, the nature of the "fellowship" as a driving force of AA compels others to think of it as a cult or religion. Buddha, Mother Nature, God, Hashem, Love, Truth, and many other names may describe an AA member's description of a Higher Power. The suggestion to choose the nature of this Higher Power is a critical freedom distinguishing it from traditional (and possibly dogmatic) religions, and it is the foundation for the spiritual nature of AA (Davis, Golie, & Jansen, 1998). It is not the type of Higher Power that is important, but the notion of human limitations and a power greater than us (Riordan & Walsh, 1994). For many, that power is within the self; a 'bigger' self that is attuned to higher values and meaning in life, rather than the 'small self' one was accustomed to. This line of thought does not require individuals to look outside themselves if that is problematic (Davis, Golie, & Jansen, 1998). For some, their Higher Power is the AA group that provides the wisdom, direction, and guidance needed for recovery. And for others, that Higher Power may be the religious God that they grew up with. Some find their Higher Power in Nature, as something that restores them to harmony and balance. Some consider the Higher Power to be their soul, and surrender themselves to its Truth and Wisdom. AA reminds their members that the steps are suggestions, not rules. One is encouraged to "turn their life over" to their chosen Higher Power and this is the cornerstone in the spiritual foundation of one's recovery.

AA is often criticized for embracing the "disease concept" also referred to as a "medical model" (Davis, Golie, & Jansen, 1998; Riordan & Walsh, 1994). Professional proponents of the strengths-based perspective may feel as though these are competing perspectives. The disease concept emphasizes the negative pathology as opposed to healthy and affirming characterizations. Providers are the experts, clients are in denial; individuals are not responsible for their condition, and the counselor identifies treatment goals. Strengths-based theory emphasizes wellness; collaborative counselor/client relationships are encouraged to design recovery plans together. Further obscuring philosophical differences, definitions of working terms are not understood; i.e., what is it that constitutes a disease? And what exactly is addiction/alcoholism? Controversy aside, the medical model has provided a means of diagnosing and treating (Davis, Golie, & Jansen, 1998). The medical 'disease' model also removes the burden of guilt from the individual without removing the responsibility for their recovery.

AA, in its pursuit of spirituality and fellowship, is criticized for fostering yet another dependence or crutch on AA itself (Riordan & Walsh, 1994). This is thought to be bad due to the American/Western notion again of independence and self-reliance. Polarizing, the AA approach which describes extreme dependence on alcohol and other drugs, advocates 'connectedness.' Connecting with others through sponsorship, fellowship, and meetings strengthens independence and does not minimize it. In other words, I think this is another case of lack of understanding about AA's approach, creating another misconception. Connectedness through AA increases independence – not dependence.

AA is criticized for requiring total abstinence "one day at a time." It is certainly not the only approach. Other approaches include acupuncture, biofeedback, pharmacology; i.e., naltrexone or antibuse, methadone maintenance, behavior modification, cognitive therapy, and solution-focused therapy (Davis, Golie, & Jansen, 1998). Abstinence is not a requirement for AA membership; only a "desire to stop." There are programs and research aimed at controlled drinking, which is opposed to the AA way of thinking. In AA, controlled drinking misses the point. The point is that if someone has found their way into an AA meeting, chances are that their drinking/drug use has long since been out of control.

Another common complaint of AA is that, probably as a result of the period the Big Book was written and AA developed, it takes on a sexist view of women. Men are commonly referred to as the alcoholic; there are not many references to the female alcoholic. The Big Book makes reference to women drinking secretively, but other references are to the woman as the alcoholics' 'spouse.' This is an example of Feminist Therapy perspective, which puts gender and power as the central issue. Feminist theory points to the social, cultural, and political context of an individual's needs (Corey, 2009). AA has responded to these concerns as demonstrated by their newer editions of *Alcoholics Anonymous.*

Some are critical of AA because they say one is forced to say, "hi, I'm _____, and I'm an alcoholic;" that this is constantly degrading and labeling (Davis, Golie, & Jansen, 1998). However, once again it is easy to miss the metaphorical significance behind AA practices. First of all, utilizing just first names, does not give significance to one's profession, family name, or where they live. It promotes anonymity, another spiritual component. Attaching "I'm an alcoholic (or addict) is what critics would call counter therapeutic or a negative label. However, for AA members this takes on the nuance of a different and positive meaning. It the context of a greeting, it carries with it a message. It implies – yes, I have faced the reality of my addiction; I am coming to terms with it; I have suffered – just like you; we understand each other; I am in recovery today pursuing physical, mental, emotional, and spiritual wellness; and I am grateful for my recovery (Davis, Golie, & Jansen, 1998).

Therefore, despite the justifications to AA philosophy, and in response to those who do not respond to AA, and in response to those who respond to other means, AA-based programs alone are few and far between. Certainly government agencies and government funded programs support and adopted a multi-faceted approach, and may even be chastised if AA is overly endorsed over other methods of recovery. The point is, in response to providing individualized care, working in collaboration with the client on treatment plans, and in an effort not to pigeonhole everyone into an AA mold, the recovery mode is left up to the client to determine what is best for them.

Comment for the Reader: I am a big fan of AA and the 12-Step process; what can I say. But, as counselors, it is important to know that it is not for everyone. Counselors who support it want to go . . ."yeah, but, but . . . !" to every discount and we tend to try to beat down whatever objection to it the client may have. What is vital, regardless of the path of recovery chosen, is that people immerse themselves in recovery. We are either moving forward toward recovery or backward toward relapse; there is no standing still. And just like they told you in Sunday school, you've got two voices talking to you. In our case, one voice is the addiction and the other is our recovery, and we need the decisional balance to be on the recovery side, and the only way to do that is to be surrounded by recovery factors; i.e., people, places, and things.

CHAPTER 12

The 12 Steps in Relation to Counseling Theories

Despite various criticisms of 12-step programs, insight into some metaphorical significance of the steps reveals parallels to the counseling theories discussed in Unit 2. Yalom and Leszcz (2005) discuss some misconceptions on the part of AA members and treatment providers alike. Some believe that 12-step groups are opposed to medication. Some get the impression the 12-step programs and philosophy somehow relinquish the member of personal responsibility. On the other side of the coin, some think that treatment programs neglect spirituality. Some feel that if they engage in a treatment program, 12-step programs are not necessary.

There are some significant differences between the 12 Step group and group therapy. A 12-Step group leader is a fellow 12-Step member. A trained professional leads group therapy. Most 12-Step groups prohibit "crosstalk," that is, specific feedback from members regarding what was shared. Group therapy thrives on that kind of feedback. Group member interaction is at the core of the group process.

In many ways, the 12 steps and group therapy approaches can complement each other. Yalom and Leszcz (2005) put the steps into secular terms that may be part of the group therapy process and/or psychotherapeutic focus. Step 1 can reflect a return to right-sized-ness, puts the problem in perspective, and releases one from unhealthy dependence. Step 1 can, in group process terms, open the door for trusting the power of the group. It utilizes existential theory; i.e., making choices and finding values. It utilizes reality theory; i.e., teaching people to take control of their life. Step 2 can set the stage for healing through relationships and connecting with the group. A "Higher Power" can be viewed as a source of comfort, peace, inner sustenance, and hope that can replace the need for drugs. Step 3 is like making a leap of faith in the recovery process. Steps 2 and 3 are also found in Jungian theory; i.e., inclusion of a Higher Consciousness as a solution. Step 4 is about looking inward for the answers. Step 5 is about sharing your secrets, sorrows, and deepest feelings as well as your joys. Steps 4 and 5 are examples of utilizing narrative therapy. Step 6 is about looking at one's internal triggers that can lead to relapse. Step 7 can be viewed as a means of accepting our behavior that interfere with fulfilling relationships, change them by learning new coping strategies, using the group as a source of insight, and as an opportunity to try new things along with a sense of self-responsibility. Steps 6 and 7 are examples in counseling of cognitive behavioral theory. Step 8 is a means of identifying persons one may have hurt in the past due to one's behavior, developing empathy for others, understanding the impact of one's actions, and gaining willingness to atone by bettering one's character. Step 8 can be correlated to Gestalt Theory and the notion of 'unfinished business.' Step 9 can be about using the group as a testing ground for what things people need to pay attention to and how to go about it. Step 9 is a study in Reality Theory and the willingness and commitment to change and follow through with one's plans. Step 10 in psychological terms can mean to become introspective, honest with oneself, and become accountable for one's behavior. Responsibility plays an integral part in Existential, Gestalt, and Reality Theory. Step 11 encourages self-soothing meditation and spiritual experience. Step 12 can be about how developing an empathic concern and care for others one can become fulfilled. Steps 11 and 12 are complimentary to person-centered concepts of actualizing one's potential.

Comment for the Reader: I like this because the 12-Step process and psychodynamics should complement each other and I like to embrace them both together. This is what a dual diagnosis paradigm is all about; that is, blending mental health and substance abuse treatment forces together in order to form pragmatic and efficacious applications to the issue. And the issue is that dual diagnosis is an antibiosis (an antagonistic association) relationship between substance abuse and mental health issues, and it is the relationship that must be treated.

CONCLUSION

The reader is encouraged to gain a working knowledge of AA. Many of its basic principles are relevant regardless of the approach to recovery taken. Unit 7 goes into this in greater detail.

In the next unit, various methods and techniques of individual and group counseling are discussed. These are basic to counseling regardless of your theoretical approach.

UNIT 3 HIGHLIGHTS

CH 11: AA Philosophy in Treatment Programs

- AA philosophy was the foundation for most treatment programs from the mid-20th century (see Chapter 4)
- AA criticisms/degrading to marginalized population/lowers self esteem/promotes religiosity – vs. – losing self to gain self/spirituality
- Disease concept vs. strengths-based model

CH 12: The 12 Steps in Relation to Counseling Theories

- The steps relinquish responsibility?
- Treatment neglects spirituality?
- 12-step practice and group counseling complement each other

STUDY GUIDE

1) Do you feel that AA philosophy belongs in treatment programs? Why? Why not?
2) What objections or reservations do you have about AA (if any)?

REFERENCES

Davis, Diane Rae, and Golie G. Jansen (1998). "Making meaning of Alcoholics Anonymous for social workers: Myths, metaphors, and realities." *Social Work* 43(2), 169-182. PsycINFO, EBSCOhost (accessed December 12, 2009).

Hugeulet, P. & Koenig, H.G. (2009). *Religion and spirituality in psychiatry.* New York: Cambridge University Press.

Mackenzie, Alisdair, and Richard P. Allen (2003). "Alcoholics' evaluations of alcoholism treatment." *Alcoholism Treatment Quarterly* 21(2), p. 1-18. PsycINFO, EBSCOhost (accessed December 12, 2009).

Ramson, R.; Obert, J.; McCann, M.; & Ling, W. (2005). Matrix Model. Center City, MN: Hazelden.

Riordan, R.; & Walsh, L. (1994). Guidelines for professional referral to Alcoholics Anonymous and other twelve-step groups. *Journal of Counseling & Development,* 72(4), 351-355. Retrieved from PsycINFO database.

Yalom, I.D. & Leszcz, M. (2005). The theory and practice of group psychotherapy. (5th ed.). NY: Basic Books.

UNIT 4/Individual and Group Counseling Skills

Introduction

The early part of this unit is devoted to a discussion about group counseling and is followed by skills that can be developed for individual counseling, and also applied in conducting groups. The chapter on motivational interviewing and stages of change is particularly relevant to the paradigm shift in the field as discussed in Chapter 10.

CHAPTER 13

Group Counseling Skills

Group counseling is the most common treatment for co-occurring disorders. It focuses on relapse prevention. Relapse prevention is about identifying triggers that cause a person to use substances, and adapting coping strategies to avoid usage.

Climate. As we get started discussing group-therapy dynamics, I think the most vital piece in group work is setting the pace by establishing the climate or tone of the group. Every so often, my group will get my 'shpiel' whether they need to hear it or not – because it's a good thing and bears repeating and reinforcing.

Particularly in substance use groups, our common purpose is one of life or death. Absolutely! And people need to be reminded of this. People die from this disease. I tell my groups that I take this very seriously and so should they. It doesn't mean that we can't have fun and laugh – because that's important, too – but no one should lose sight of the fact that if they are sitting in this group (Intensive Outpatient), they have earned their seat here (to borrow an expression from AA). I want people to know and understand that most importantly, I want them to feel safe in a group. One of my clients told me that this (the group) is where the magic happens! And that is only possible if we set, have, and maintain the right atmosphere for people to feel comfortable enough to put whatever they have to – out there – and to do so without any fear of breach of confidentiality, or fear of not being respected. I let people know that hostile or threatening behavior of any kind will not be tolerated. I tell them that I do what I do because I have found that things you don't think are possible – can be possible – and I want them to know that.

I believe that because my tone is genuine, hopeful, and serious, and because I mean business right from the get go, people in the group (or at least many in it) are able to adopt a trusting, if not tentative, approach to the group. It is up to the facilitator to set the pace and provide the group with the confidence that the tone will be maintained.

Group Work. In most behavioral health treatment programs, including mental health groups, substance abuse groups, and dual-diagnosis groups, groups are ongoing, continual, and open-ended. In other words, the group does not usually start together and finish together. Typically, there are new people coming in all the time, as well as those who have completed their program and are being discharged. Thus, there is a round-robin type of effect. Groups are often described by beginning, middle, and end stages; and the ongoing group has its own set of advantages and disadvantages. This overview is by no means a comprehensive review of group process, but will provide the early counselor with some basic tenets involved in group work.

Early Stages. There are characteristics of the group process, however, which may be applicable to either type of group. The early stages for the group or the individual new member carry certain common experiences.

This is always a time for introductions – ongoing groups are going to do this frequently as new members join the group, as opposed to members who have been with the group since its inception. And in any group, it is wise to remind people of any group rules, housekeeping details, the purpose of the group, and its agenda. (Jacobs, Masson, & Harvill, 2009). It may take the new member two or three sessions before their trust and comfort level becomes productive. Garland, Jones and Kolodny (1973) call this pre-affiliation, that is, a stage when members become acclimated to the group. A range of emotions may be experienced; both fear and hope, uneasiness and anticipation. They may need to see the group in operation before testing the waters (Jacobs, Masson, & Harvill, 2009; Yalom & Leszcz, 2005). What is the tone of the group? How much will they really be able to put out there? What kind of response are they going to get? Typically, they will look to the group leader for guidance rather than other group members before hopefully finding common ground, acceptance, respect, and approval (Jacobs, Masson, & Harvill, 2009; Yalom & Leszcz, 2005). It is only then that members may experiment with new behaviors (Yalom & Leszcz, 2005). Any attempts by the counselor to ease new members' anxiety are usually beneficial (Yalom & Leszcz, 2005). Everyone has a purpose for being in the group and there is also a need to find their niche in the group, and this involves their social relationships with other members of the group (Jacobs, Masson, & Harvill, 2009). Inevitably, members size each other up. Some members will be defensive and some may become dominant, but most are particularly vulnerable at this point. Most will have a deep-seated need for a one-to-one connection, as well as a connection with the group (Yalom & Leszcz, 2005). As a result, group members will look to the group leader for structure, expectations, direction, and care (Jacobs, Masson, & Harvill, 2009; Yalom & Leszcz, 2005). What does this mean for the new counselor? Each counselor will develop their own style that they are comfortable with. I do think though, that it is important for the counselor to possess a good sense of themselves and understand they are a role model for their clients. This does not mean they must conceal their vulnerabilities. It does mean they must have integrity about them. In other words, you can be who you are, but you must be authentic about it because clients will sense anything less and they will respect your honesty, appreciate your sincerity, and identify with your humanness, whether or not they agree with you or like you.

Power and Control. Yalom and Leszcz (2005) (p. 314) make note of the social hierarchy that develops in the group. There are invariably, struggles for power, control, and dominance, and a "preferred amount of initiative." This stage can include scapegoating, certain resentment and anger that may be aimed at the group leader, and the group leader's counter transference as well. Members go from deciding if they belong in the group to being concerned about their rank in the group. Groups within the group may form for support. There are, no doubt, isolated members who fall to the periphery of the group. Many members struggle with relating and engaging with the group.

Largely, the counselor lets these things play out; it is not possible to control all these different elements. However, the counselor must be a fulcrum and keep the group on its primary purpose and on task. The counselor needs to listen to their instincts – this is why you do what you do. If you sense someone is being scapegoated, address it. If you sense someone is being left out or not connecting, address it. If you sense that everyone is avoiding an issue, address it. Sometimes, it is as though the group has a headache and can't do much else until it gets relieved.

Working Stage. Once past finding their place in the group, Jacobs, Masson, and Harvill (2009) state that members begin to focus on why they are there. This is called the working stage, is central to group progress, and hopefully it is when the members start to experience benefits from being a part of the group (Jacobs, Masson, & Harvill, 2009). A good working group will develop cohesion (Yalom & Leszcz, 2005). People may disclose more – there is safety, trust, rapport, affinity, and kinship. This may be interrupted at times when older members of the group are discharged and new members are admitted. The group will need to rebalance itself and deepen its personal involvement and value in the group (Jacobs, Masson, & Harvill, 2009; Yalom & Leszcz, 2005). Yalom & Leszcz, (2005) describe cohesion. Group moral can grow when older members begin to make some progress and become models for newer members of the group. There can be greater freedom of expression and acceptance as people get to know each other better. The group takes on an identity and it becomes a strong viable part of members' lives. Members become skilled at working through problems and begin to rely on the group for support and feedback. The group leader facilitates, supports, guides, and directs the group and keeps it focused on task.

Discharge. This period represents the end of the group for the group member. They have completed their program and now it is time to move on, perhaps to aftercare or into the community. They are now separating from the group (Jacobs, Masson, & Harvill, 2009). They may have become a leader in the group and like the opportunity to share what they have learned. They may have begun to pull away and become less involved. Often members who were reluctant to join the group now do not want to leave, and it can be an emotional time (Jacobs, Masson, & Harvill, 2009; Yalom & Leszcz, 2005).

Group Pitfalls. There are obstacles and problems that face any group. As indicated with the on-going group, there is a constant turnover. The group leader and the group must be able to absorb this. A very strong, but underestimated factor in the group, is the impact that each member has on the group. Excessive absences or tardiness affect the group in terms of interruptions and consistency. One member's relapse is going to be felt throughout the group. Clients may be surprised, disappointed, and angry, and have a heightened sense of their own vulnerability. Clients can wind up going to jail, which is the epitome of many members' fears. Clients may just drop out and not be heard from again; this can tear at the fabric of the group's cohesiveness. There may be times when a member needs to be asked to leave. Hostile and threatening behavior cannot be tolerated. Perhaps they are in non-compliance for continued substance use. Whatever the reason, it will no doubt have great impact for the member and the group. Sometimes confidentiality issues prevent the group leader from disclosing the details. The group may surmise the circumstances, but is often left to wonder.

Cliques can form. New members may be excluded. Sub-groups can develop in response to group conflicts of various natures (Yalom & Leszcz, 2005). There can be motivation differences, resentments, personality conflicts, and gender issues. There can be conflicts that arise in therapy, and hostilities that arise. There are termination issues (Yalom & Leszcz, 2005). Often, the group will have at least one 'difficult' member. Let's take a look.

Difficult Group Members

The Central Character. The first difficult member worth discussing is what I call the 'Central Character.' These folks, either by incessant talking, or by a need to dominate the group, manage to monopolize the group's time. Some nervous members talk a lot in order to hide their feelings or in an effort to try to control their feelings. Some just ramble on and on and don't realize what they are doing; they are just verbose individuals. Some persons want to impress the group leader or show the group how much they know (Jacobs, Masson & Harvill, 2009).

In any of these cases, a number of things occur. Certain other members may be relieved that they are not the focus of attention and are perfectly willing to let this person continue in their role. Silent clients can also be a problem. Research demonstrates that the more members participate, the greater their sense of change (Yalom & Leszcz, 2005). Others may get angry and resent this individual. There are a couple of ways to handle the situation. First of all, sometimes this individual's dominance of the group may be a smokescreen to hide what is really going on for them (Yalom & Lesczcz, 2005). The group might actually focus more attention on this individual to get at their core issues. At other times, it may be necessary to speak with the client privately to save embarrassment. It can be done in the group as well, but tactfully.

The Pain in the Neck. I say that affectionately, but some clients can be more difficult to work with than others. We often have clients who are a distraction or annoyance to the group. They seem to get the group off track, or inadvertently do things that detract the focus of the group. Sometimes an Attention Deficit client or Hyperactive client cannot sit still or quietly for long. Other clients seem to vie for attention of any kind. Talking with the member may not actually help; albeit then ignoring their comments or behavior may not help, either (Jacobs, Masson, & Harvill, 2009). If a client's behavior is disruptive to the point of intruding on other members, they may be asked to leave. Hostile and/or threatening behavior is never acceptable, and the client may be asked to leave because the safety of the group comes first. There are times when this needs to be done immediately; otherwise, it may be best to wait till the end of the group and done privately to avoid a power struggle in front of the group.

The Helper. Often, members try to rescue each other (Jacobs, Masson, & Harvill, 2009; Yalom & Leszcz, 2005). This is well intended and can feel like it is adding to the cohesion of the group. And it may, but the problem is that the client who is in pain may just need to be listened to and supported, and does not need guidance, recommendations, or understanding. The group leader can simply redirect the group (Jacobs, Masson, & Harvill, 2009). Also, the helper is often just taking focus off of themselves.

The Nay-Sayer. The client with the negative attitude can be a problem (Jacobs, Masson, & Harvill, 2009; Yalom & Leszcz, 2005). They can create a negative climate and even gain allies. They can interfere with group goals and cohesion, and they can make it difficult for the counselor. Generally speaking, the counselor does not want to confront this member in group because it can turn into an argument, which first of all doesn't feel good, and is going to be unproductive (Jacobs, Masson, & Harvill, 2009). It's tempting for the counselor to address the issues in group but it can turn into a struggle for power. It may be best to speak with this member outside of the group to try to determine why they are so negative (Jacobs, Masson & Harvill, 2009).

Along the same lines, particularly in substance abuse groups, many clients may be forced to be there; i.e., or face legal consequences. They, too, can create a negative environment that is not conducive to the safe and trusting tone needed. They either don't want to be there; don't think that they need to, don't believe the group is going to help, or otherwise do not want to change. Sometimes spending too much time with this client can take away from the productiveness of the group. Pick your battles. Jacobs, Masson & Harvill (2009) stress, "don't unzip the client unless you can zip him back up (p. 345)." (I love that!) that can require strong individual counseling skills. However, providing a safe atmosphere for all members to feel comfortable to share is a priority for the group leader; I do not tolerate one (or more) members disrupting the group in that fashion. If their conduct or manner is having a negative impact on the group, they may be asked to leave. It is one thing to not want to be in the group and it is another to interfere with other group members getting what they came for.

Psychiatric Clients. There is what I like to call 'soft' diagnoses like anxiety and depression, and then there are 'hard' diagnoses like bipolar disorder, schizophrenia, and certain personality disorders. Not that anxiety and/or depression cannot be truly debilitating, but a psychotic, delusional, manic client or a fellow walking to the beat of his own drum may be particularly difficult to deal with. This is not to say, by any means, that they cannot grasp recovery (I know many who understand why they need to be abstinent and enjoy years of sobriety), but many face much greater obstacles than the one-dimensionally diagnosed client (Pray & Watson, 2008). Furthermore, dual diagnosed clients' quality of life is poorer than the one-dimensionally diagnosed client (Henson, 2008). In the group, their symptoms may be a distraction. The counselor cannot let the group run amuck; it is a terrible feeling. Whatever the distraction, how it detracts from the group purpose can usually be discussed and helps to refocus the group.

I wish to digress for a moment with another word about harm reduction at this juncture (see Chapter 6). Most of the time, treatment programs' primary focus is relapse prevention and the primary goal is abstinence. But, this is not always the case. The notion of "harm reduction" is often met with bewilderment and confusion, and is provocative and controversial, as well. You will recall, harm reduction is defined as 1) reducing the frequency of drug usage and/or 2) reducing the harmful consequences that result from drug usage (MacMaster, 2004). Some of you are no doubt still cringing. I did, too. It sounds like a tacit approval to use, doesn't it? But I assure you, there is a place for this line of thinking in current treatment methods. Consider the chronic relapser, with over a couple of dozen inpatient hospitalizations and as many outpatient programs. If abstinence is the only measuring stick for treatment, chances are this is going to be a setup for failure and another blow to their esteem. If they can be taught greater skills that help them increase the length of time between usage, or not be involved in as much criminal activity, or not contract a serious and communicable disease, that is a good thing! Needle exchange programs, pamphlets that show addicts how to use "in a safer way," and methadone maintenance programs are all examples of harm reduction. The addict we are describing may be a chronic relapser for a couple of reasons. They may have cognitive difficulties that increase the chance of relapse. Then there is the addict who just simply doesn't want to stop. Many times we take a harm reduction approach to the psychiatric client. In the group, the counselor wants to engage him/her; we don't want them walking out the door. The simple, short answer is that we use their own strengths, feeling, thoughts, and insights to help them make better decisions that move them forward toward their goals and desires in life.

Dealing with Silence. This can be a nightmare for the beginner counselor – when nobody says anything, what to do? The impulse for most, is to take matters into their own hands and say something to get the conversation going again. Jacobs, Masson, and Harvill (2009) might disagree, but I would say: Resist the urge. Resist the urge until you have an inkling why the group is quiet.

If the group is new, or there are several new members that have changed the dynamics of the group, group members may be fearful not knowing what is expected or what to do. To perpetuate the silence in this case, will probably create confusion.

There are other times, however, when members of the group need to wrestle with their roles in the group and their purpose in being there. Many times, the group can become quiet and no one wants to assume responsibility. Eventually, there's always one or two who are too uncomfortable with the silence and feel the need to say something. The group is the group's responsibility. The group leader should not be doing all the work and the group members need to have a sense of responsibility to themselves and to each other for what happens in the group. The group leader is the group's 'facilitator'

. . . that means to make the process easier; they assist but are not the producer of the end result. It is not suggested that the facilitator let the silence to go on indefinitely because that may become counter-productive, but certainly long enough to allow members' an opportunity to think about what they will do or not do about the quiet.

Group Cohesion. A good sense of responsibility to the group can help to generate a good sense of cohesiveness in the group (Yalom & Leszcz, 2005). It's like glue. The group tends to stick together when they are working well together and when they have a common purpose or goal. This can be easier for a substance abuse group because everyone is there for the same reason. Even if a member does not want to stop using or is not ready to, or if he/she is in a legal situation, it is going to be in their interest to stop using long enough until the crisis, situation, or consequences go away. And that is a perfectly acceptable position. The common goal is to stop using drugs. The common purpose is to learn to enjoy life without the use of drugs. A treatment group becomes like a lifeboat and everyone needs to work together to get to shore. Yalom and Leszcz (2005) liken cohesion in the group to the therapeutic alliance that emerges in individual counseling. It is an essential ingredient.

Furthermore, with a substance abuse group, those who are into 12-Step meetings will bring back the feeling of fellowship. Narcotics Anonymous is known as a "we" program. Remember, just like the individual counselor wants to create that therapeutic climate with client, they want to keep the group's environment with the same working atmosphere. It should not be taken for granted and the group leader must always be sensitive to things that threaten that environment. Many things can threaten the therapeutic climate, such as an unmotivated new member, an argument between two members, an unexpected administrative discharge (perhaps for poor attendance or behavior), a member unexpectedly going to jail or inpatient, or so forth. The group leader must always try to bring the group back and periodically remind the group of its common purpose and the importance of having a safe environment in the group where everyone can feel secure enough to talk about whatever they may need to. As a result of common purpose, there are certain factors the group underscores and strives to achieve. These are referred to as curative factors.

> *Comment for the Reader:* You know, working with groups is very exciting and I've come to enjoy it more than individual work. I am very grateful to Irving Yalom in *Love's Executioner*, who freely shares about resisting the urge to fall asleep during boring individual therapy sessions! Group work is extremely dynamic and can be immensely powerful. Just like you have "Aha!" moments in individual therapy, in group therapy there are moments when the group is swept over with intense emotion simultaneously – when everyone is on the same page of that experience. It is moving and profound for all and serves to solidify the group. And, if you know me, I will always take the opportunity to let people know that what they are experiencing in the group – they can find in AA. "The group" can be a special and esoteric experience for many and I think it's very important for them to know they can experience it in the community – the fellowship that is.

CHAPTER 14

YALOM'S CURATIVE FACTORS

Remedial Group Influences. A good working cohesive group thrives on a set of influences that provide meaning and purpose for group members. Yalom and Leszcz (2005) purport 11 therapeutic factors that are curative in nature.

The first is the instillation of hope or the belief that the group is going to somehow help to relieve their burden. Hope and faith are spiritual factors and there is a plethora of research that demonstrates that spirituality is associated with wellness and quality of life (Galanter, 2005; Temple University, 2009; Han, 2009; Liberman, 2008; Heintzman, 2008; Delgado, 2007; Cole & Pargament, 1999; Dein & Stygal, 1997; Koenig, 1997; Pargament, 1997; Pargament, Smith, Koenig, & Perez, 1998). If the client has made it to your group, to borrow an AA expression, they have most likely "earned their seat." They may well be beaten down by the disease physically, emotionally, and spiritually not to mention legal and family complications, broken relationships, and ravaged lives. All that many people have left is some linger of hope.

The second factor is universality; that is, the fact that they are not alone. Many addicts/alcoholics have been driven into emotional isolation (if not physical isolation, as well). People feel alone in their mire of shame and circumstance. It is a tremendous relief to discover that others have been hiding in the shadows of a broken and ruined self as well. People embrace each other's acts of immorality with understanding and compassion. They are "home" in the group and become closer to other members than their own family. Certainly no one can be made to fully understand the addict's experience, except those who have lived it. The NA preamble states that "the therapeutic act of one addict helping another is without parallel" (Narcotics Anonymous, 1984, p. 16).

The next factor is the imparting of information. Members can gain viable insight into their specific triggers to drug/drink as well as learning some real strategies to avoid the drug/drink. Programs today are centered around teaching a variety of cognitive behavioral therapy solution-focused skills not to mention common themes in addiction/alcoholism, including the medical and learning models as well as 12-Step model. Information is abundant and members have an opportunity to practice new behaviors in groups.

Altruism is another curative force. People gain by giving. This is at the heart of the 12-Step process. AA's 12th Step is about "carrying the message" of recovery. It seems to be an essential ingredient; there is an intrinsic value to giving. It sustains group cohesion. The group leader may direct and steer the group, but members often find the backing, reassurance, recommendations, and insights from other group members more desirable and valuable.

Groups offer members an opportunity to experience a setting that resembles the mechanics and forces of the structure of a family. The group leader is often like a mother or father and there is a certain transference to this authority figure. The other group members can be like brothers and sisters. This type of group process surfaces and reveals many assumptions, including irrational and faulty thinking, unfinished business, and experiences the member may have had with their family, in a way that individual counseling cannot. When discussed with the group, they can be corrected and begin to lose their stigma and impact.

The group can provide the opportunity to model behavior learned from the counselor as well as other group members. Examples may be a steady, confident, business- like approach to tackling problems, or the ability to self-disclose or provide support. The group provides a chance to reinforce new coping methods, new ways of expressing themselves, and an opportunity to be the new person they have grown into.

Groups provide an invaluable opportunity to interact with others. Members can practice interpersonal skills in their new relationships. The group can provide, through the relationships that develop, a milieu where the member can gain the means to handle what previously was an unmanageable experience. The group is ideally a safe place for some risk taking. After some time, members are able to relax and be themselves with other group members. What this does is to reveal maladaptive behaviors. Individual styles and conduct become manifest to the group and there is no need for the member to explain themselves, as it has become evident and become the business of the group.

Group cohesion is Yalom and Leszcz (2005) ninth curative factor and was previously discussed. Perhaps as a result of the previous therapeutic forces, the member is able to discuss things in group they may never have been able to discuss in the past. This type of cathartic experience is often believed to be of great value. Yalom and Leszcz (2005) indicate that while it is testimony to the effectiveness of all of the curative factors, sharing is not indicative of change. However, change is better indicated when the sharing is linked with cognitive learning.

It is interesting to note that in a study conducted by Lese and McNair-Semands (2000), twenty long-term group therapy members rated the twelve categories of curative factors outlined herein and the number-one-valued item in group therapy was "discovering and accepting previously unknown or unacceptable parts of me" (Yalom & Leszcz, 2005, p. 85). Furthermore, these insights often concerned positive aspects they learned about themselves.

The last therapeutic factor identified describes the member's ability to accept responsibility for themselves and their lives. Imbedded in this category are several factors. There is recognition that life can be unfair and that there is no escaping it. There is recognition that regardless of the people in one's life, ultimately life is faced alone. There is now an effort to live in a more honest way, because, despite help and support from others, ultimately one is responsible for the way one lives.

> *Comment for the Reader:* These are cool. The curative factors are why groups work; this is what people get from participating in a group. If you understand why these factors are essential and work, then you are at the heart of the matter.

CHAPTER 15

THERAPIST COMMUNICATION SKILLS

We have discussed various objectives of different therapeutic approaches. This next section will outline effective counselor skills when working with clients that are useful with all theoretical orientations. Common goals of therapy are questioning, understanding, and problem-solving. Presented here are several methods of communicating with clients that assist in those goals. They apply to both individual and group counseling.

The first is called attending or active listening (Okun, 2002). This is about simply paying attention to the client. It involves listening to what the client is saying as well as to their voice; being aware of body language, eye contact, sitting attentively; and letting the client know you are listening (Corey, 2009). For example, perhaps the client's voice is cracking while they are speaking to you; are their arms and legs folded or crossed; are they turned away from you; do they avoid looking at you? This applies to individual and group therapy, except that in a group the counselor scans the group catching nonverbal cues, facial expressions and body language (Jacobs, Masson & Harvill, 2009). The occasional nod or 'yes' or 'I see' is affirming to the client (Okun, 2002).

There are various ways of responding to the client, and the first is called paraphrasing. This is when the counselor repeats what the client has said using different words. This lets the client know we are listening (Okun, 2002). Reflecting is a little different; it adds an understanding of the client's effect. In other words, the counselor communicates their sense of the client's implied feelings. The therapist checks what is not being said, what the client is emphasizing, or a shift in posture. Reflection lets the client know we are not only listening, but understanding. (Okun, 2002; Corey, 2009). Sometimes the client gives us a complicated, jumbled, or vague message. When counselors are unsure of what the client has said, they check their understanding with the client so both are on the same page (Okun, 2002).

For example . . .

Client: ". . . so I explained to him (her father) . . . that I couldn't pay the mortgage . . . (voice raised and quivering).

Therapist (paraphrasing): ". . . you told your dad you didn't have any money and couldn't pay your bills."

Therapist (reflective): ". . . it upset you that you don't have enough money and had to tell your dad. . . ."

Counselors will sometimes question or probe the client. Your theoretical orientation will determine what type of questions you may ask. Questions that encourage the client to explore ideas and develop insight into themselves are different than probing for information. Questions will be open-ended as opposed to seeking a definitive answer.

For example . . .

Open-ended: "How did you feel when asked for a divorce?" "What did you think when she told you she was alcoholic?"

Closed-ended: "Where did you go to school?" "Are you employed?"

The Gestalt and Reality therapist will probably not ask 'why' questions. Rational Emotive Therapy will use questions frequently to help the client examine irrational thinking (Corey, 2009; Okun, 2002).

Interpretation takes reflection a step further. Psychoanalysts use interpretation to let the client know what the underlying meaning may be to their thoughts, feelings, and behavior. Of course, we can be wrong! Or, we may give the client information they are not ready for, or the client may become reliant on us to figure things out (Corey, 2009). The Gestalt approach helps the clients make their own interpretations. Remember, person-centered therapy has faith in the individual's ability to figure things out for themselves within the right atmosphere. Sometimes, though, interpreting can be useful to the client's understanding (Corey, 2009; Okun, 2002).

For example (see paraphrasing and reflective examples) . . .

Therapist (interpretative): ". . . it was humiliating to have to tell dad you couldn't pay the mortgage. . . ."

Summarizing on the part of the counselors can help the client put all their thoughts and feelings together. It combines the various things they've been saying, putting their feelings, ideas, and subjects into a common theme or themes. The counselor will highlight certain aspects in order to further clarify what is being said. It can be a way of summing a session or recapping last week, or when a client rapidly brings up a lot of issues – it can be a way of narrowing things down (Okun, 2002). Summarizing is an important skill in group work. Many viewpoints may be stated. It may be a way of concluding what someone has said who has been speaking for a while. Summarizing can be a way of ending one discourse and moving on to something else. (Jacobs, Masson, & Harvill, 2009). Along this line the counselor may link what one person has said to another's statement, thereby tying things together. This can be a good way for members to bond and feel connected (Jacobs, Masson & Harvill, 2009).

For example . . .

Therapist (summarizing): ". . . last week you were telling me how you lost your job and you went out drinking . . . and this week, you're upset about having to talk to dad about money. . . . I see all this is difficult to cope with. . . ."

Both in group therapy and individual counseling, supporting and reassurance are a part of every theoretical orientation (Corey, 2009). Supporting comments let the client know that you have heard and understood what they said and that it is not unusual (Okun, 2002). Encouragement assists the client through their anxiety, frustration, or concerns to move forward. Person-centered therapy is all about setting the right supportive atmosphere (Corey, 2009). Especially in group, clients are concerned with how they appear to others. The counselor wants to communicate warmth and reassurance to give the client a sense of confidence about taking a risk (Jacobs, Masson & Haverill, 2009). The counselor may often express approval by statements, which agree with the client.

For example . . .

Therapist (supportive): ". . . you've always been so resourceful in the past, I know you'll find a way to work through this, too!"

Along the same lines, the counselor will need to set the tone for the group – that is, create the mood. We discussed creating a climate in the chapter on groups. This is very important. A few encouraging and caring words about sharing, trusting, and confidentiality can establish a positive atmosphere (Jacobs, Masson & Haverill, 2009).

Related to tone and support is confrontation. Confrontation is never done in an adversarial way, but is a sincere and constructive challenge. If the right atmosphere has been established the relationship will endure the confrontation individually or in a group (Okun, 2002). It is never an attack but an invitation to take a look at an issue from another perspective (Corey, 2009). It may involve pointing out a discrepancy or inconsistency in what the client is saying or doing in an effort to look at an issue more honestly.

For example . . .

Therapist (confrontational): ". . . I know these are tough times, but in the past you've used that as an excuse to let your drinking get out of control. . . ."

One more aspect to our communications with a client is that of informing or instructing. Providing information is to be distinguished from giving advice. Providing factual information allows the clients to formulate their own decision. Advice can be okay, but it is subjective and verges on telling the client what to do (Okun, 2002). What's wrong with that? Remember, there has been that paradigm shift in therapy from the counselor as 'expert' to placing that responsibility on the client. Why? It helps the client become autonomous and to begin relying on themselves for the answers.

For example . . .

Therapist (as expert): ". . . you need to get back to AA meetings right away. . . ."

Therapist (as collaborator): ". . . I know you've been through this before . . . what's worked for you in the past?"

Do you see how different these can feel?

Transference and Counter-Transference

A word about transference and counter-transference is appropriate in this section about individual and group interactions with our clients. We have all heard about these concepts. Transference is central to the helping relationship; it occurs when the client infers emotions and attitudes they have from their parent-child relationships to the therapist (Okun, 2002). Okun (2002) cites Watkins (1983) regarding roles attributed to the counselor through transference as "the ideal, the seer, the nurturer, the frustrater, or the non-entity." The perspective the client has regarding the counselor will help determine what expectations they about him/her. Feelings toward the counselor resulting from transference may be love, sexual, hostile, anxious, resentful. The counselor may be seen as an authority figure who can punish, demand, or control (Corey, 2009). Transference can represent an opportunity to resolve conflicts through the model the counselor represents. It also presents insights about how the client responds to present relationships based on past relationships (Okun, 2002).

Counter-transference is when the client elicits sources of conflicts on the part of the counselor. This can be both positive and negative. The danger for the counselor is that they personalize their unresolved feelings onto the client. The counselor may need to work through it in order to provide objective care to the client (Okun, 2002). The counselor must be aware how their conflicts can be triggered by the client. Counselors must be aware of their own vulnerabilities that may intrude from time to time (Corey, 2009).

SELF-DISCLOSURE

Corey (2009) presents a good discussion about self-disclosure. There is a common misconception among beginner counselors that they need to be passive and just listen and reflect. Some of this is 'old school' derived from psychoanalytic therapy. But often, the beginner counselor wonders about their speculations and if they should say something or not. I said early on that your instincts are probably pretty good; you have to learn to trust your intuition. The trick about self-disclosure is to ask yourself, "who will benefit by the disclosure?" Is it going to make you, the counselor, feel good, or is it going to help the client? So at this juncture, some counselors either share too little or too much.

The client does wonder what your reactions are to them and does want to know what you are thinking about them during the session, as well as how you think they are doing. Some counselors focus too much on the client, questioning and probing, wanting the client to open up and become aloof and the client is then left wondering 'what's going on with you'!

At the other end of things, some counselors want to show the client how human and relatable they are – sometimes too much is revealed and the counselor becomes the focus of the session.

Usually with a few words and a confiding look, the counselor can convey understanding. If the disclosure is directly related to the client's issue at hand, it may be useful. The disclosure should not be rehearsed and mechanical, but arise spontaneously so that it is an authentic response.

At some point, every substance abuse counselor gets asked whether or not they are in recovery. For those who are recovering, some are comfortable revealing their history and some are not. It's your choice. Typically, however, those who are not in recovery deflect the question and say something like, "why is it important to you?" Many professionals advocate for this approach because the counselor can then respond directly to what the concern is. The client may say something like . . . "well, I'd like to work with someone who has been through it and knows what he's talking about". . . and this may be an intimidating question for a new counselor. However you respond, be authentic – be real! Authenticity, genuineness, caring, and a therapeutic alliance are the essential ingredients for counseling dual clients, not whether or not you are recovering.

On the other hand, I think deflecting the question can be an impersonal answer and clients can resent the fact that you won't answer the question! Answer the question! Draw on your sense of your self and strong inclination to this field. You do not have to say you are in recovery or not in recovery to convey your compassion, concern, desire, and ability to help.

I think the important thing here is that the question get dealt with on a genuine and authentic level. First of all, we as counselors need to be comfortable enough with who we are to stand on who we are. This doesn't mean you must disclose, but you do need to be comfortable with your decision about it and how you handle the issue. In other words, whatever your position is, respond in a real way.

Let me just say that whether you are in Recovery yourself or not is not a prerequisite to being a good counselor. Many clients express preference for the recovering addict/alcoholic – but that is not a guarantee of effectiveness. I think the real concern is how well we establish a therapeutic relationship or alliance with the client; this is what really determines our effectiveness.

CHAPTER 16

The Stages of Change and Motivational Interviewing

The Stages of Change, developed by Prochaska, Norcross, and DiClemente (1994) and Motivational Interviewing, developed by Miller and Rollnick (1991) go hand in hand with Rogers' humanistic person-centered therapy. Rogers affirmed that clients have the capacity within themselves to find their own answers and to actualize their potential given the right environment. The stages of change represent a framework for a continuum of phases that individuals experience when growing and changing (Prochaska & Norcross, 2001). Motivational interviewing is a technique that can gently assist the client through that continuum (Miller & Rollnick, 1991).

We shall discuss five basic stages that people pass through when undergoing change (Prochaska, Norcross & DiClemente, 1994; Prochaska & Norcross, 2001). They are precontemplation, contemplation, preparation, action, and maintenance. Think about your clients or people you know as we describe the stages.

Precontemplation. Precontemplation is the first stage. At this point, there is no desire or plan to change. There is not yet a real awareness that there is a problem indicating change is necessary. In most cases, there may be external pressures coming from the courts, family services, employers, family, or friends. This individual does not intend to change at this time nor are they seriously considering change.

Contemplation. In this stage, people have become aware that there is a problem and have begun to think about doing something about it, but have made no commitment to do so. People can be in this stage for a long time. There can be a lot of reasons why people are not ready to make any changes at this point. They may be postponing a decision based on bad information (i.e., pot is not addictive). They may have thus made a personal choice to tolerate negative consequences as a result of their using. They may be in denial and not yet see the truth.

There can be both a fear of failing and a fear of succeeding. What would one do if they stopped using?

Preparation. Now the client is beginning to think about change, but maybe unsure how to go about it. They may have had unsuccessful attempts in the past. Maybe they have reduced their usage; they do not yet have a plan. This individual wants to change at this point.

Action. Clients have started to make changes here and are motivated to work. There are overt behavior changes and there is a relative commitment to put the time and energy into it.

Maintenance. At this point, the client has achieved abstinence for an extended period (maybe 6 months) and works on preventing relapse. They have begun to experience the benefits of abstinence and do not want to lose their gains.

I have seen two other stages indicated, depending on whom you read. One is 'relapse;' this is when, obviously, a client starts using substances after a period of abstinence. Not an unlikely scenario; relapse is often a part of the process. Also, it should be noted that these stages are not always a hierarchy or even a vertical climb. Many vacillate between stages, which I like to think of more in terms of a continuum. Some list termination as the final stage when the individual has completed the change process. But, I'm not sure we do ever complete the change process; it's my experience that we always must have a certain vigilance and should never be so confident in our efficacy to deal with high risk situations. There may be zero temptation, but let's not underestimate this 'cunning, baffling, and powerful' disease, right?

Let's move on to motivational interviewing (MI) and then take a look at how it is used in conjunction with the stages of change. According to Scherling (2004), MI operates on certain assumptions about motivation. Motivation is a key to change, is multidimensional, is a dynamic and fluctuating state, is interactive, is changeable and can be modified; and lastly, is actively influenced by the helping relationship.

Keeping in mind our person-centered paradigm and strengths-based model, the basic strategies of MI are as follows. According to Scherling (2004), when working with the client, the counselor focuses on strengths rather than problems. The counselor must always respect the client's independence and the right and ability to make their own decisions. In an attempt not to depersonalize the client, problem-based diagnoses are not used. MI is based on a therapeutic partnership; the counselor is a source of information and a tool – not the 'expert, director, or final authority.' When working with the client, the counselor uses empathy and negotiation not power, or control. The counselor wishes to engage the client wherever the client is in order to prevent them from leaving prematurely. We don't get to work with the client if they get turned off and leave. The counselor must think of the stages of change as a continuum for change, not a hierarchy of categories. People move back and forth throughout early recovery. The counselor must remember that the majority of clients today are dual-diagnosis and are struggling with more than one issue. Treatment steps involved in various stages of change may be innovative, short term, and incremental.

Consistent with a person-centered approach, let's look at the skills a counselor will use to conduct MI. Scherling (2004) indicates that first and foremost the counselor employs a perspective of empathy and reflective listening. They must convey a sense of respect, acceptance, and nonjudgment for the individual's thoughts, feelings, and decisions, and develop a supportive and collaborative working alliance with the client. The counselor's role is being a resource to the client. The counselor commends the client and strengthens them; does not criticize, degrade, or shame. The counselor listens; does not tell. The counselor uses gentle persuasion by exemplifying discrepancies between the client's goals and present actions, but allows the client the room to make their own decisions. The counselor continues to support the client through the change process and avoids arguing points, and confrontation. The counselor learns to roll with the client's resistance by adjusting their approach; they do not fight with or oppose the client. The counselor believes in the client's innate ability to uncover answers themselves and remains optimistic about outcomes.

Scherling (2004) describes strategies to be employed when talking with the client: reflective listening, open-ended questions, affirmations, summarizations, and facilitate statements impelling change. As discussed earlier, reflective listening is a method of checking with the client what they are saying or mean. The counselor rewords and repeats what they understood the client to be saying. Open-ended are questions calling for a response rather than a simple 'yes' or 'no.' Usually 'why,' 'what,' and 'how' questions can elicit a thoughtful answer. We want the client to do most of the talking; we provide the supportive, accepting, trustful atmosphere for them to do so. The counselor may provide positive affirmations to the client; commending and praising, showing appreciation for their efforts and an understanding of the client's thoughts and feelings. The counselor provides summarizing statements to tie things together. It is the clients who actually present their own arguments for change. For example, if the daily opiate user expresses a desire to go to college, there is then a discrepancy between their goals and present capacity. We do not attempt to attack the client's denial; this only makes the client defend the fact that he does have a problem. Instead, the counselor builds on any clients' remarks suggesting recognition of a problem, expressing their concerns, indications of a desire to change, and optimism about change. If a client does not come to you, one way to facilitate these types of statements is to ask for them. Problem recognition: What consequences have there been as a result of your using? Are there more? Expressions of concern: What were your thoughts about that? What else? Desire to change: What do you think would the pros of changing? Can you think of other reasons? Expressing optimism: What strengths do you have that you could use if you decided to change? What's worked for you in the past? The counselor can always encourage the client to elaborate on their statements.

There are other techniques (Schering, 2004). One is having the client fill in a decisional grid. On one side of a piece of paper, have the client list all the pros and cons of continuing to use drugs/alcohol; on the other side, have them list all the pros and cons of making a change. Another method is to have the client look at extremes; i.e., what is the worst thing that could happen if you continue to use? Or, have the client look back at life before using – and now – and compare. And have the client look forward. If you were to change, what are your hopes for the future? The counselor may employ paradoxical therapy. Take the position that drugs are not a problem. This can induce the client into sharing their concerns and conflicts about continuing to use. Also, you can use good-hearted humor as well, taken right from the client's own experiences.

Stagework. The counselor has goals for each stage of change. When the client is in a precontemplative stage, the best thing the counselor can do is establish a therapeutic alliance. Try to bring out awareness of the client's situation; i.e, the consequences as a result of drug use. Tap into any hint of the client's doubt that the substance use may not be harmless. Help the clients look down the road to determine for themselves where their behavior is taking them. When the client is in the contemplation stage, play off of the client's ambivalence about continuing to use. Talk about the external motivation that may exist;

i.e., familial, occupational, or legal ramifications. Work on internal motivation by having the client look at where he is and where he wants to go. When preparing to change, the counselor assists the client in strengthening their commitment to change and to develop confidence about their ability to accomplish their goals. The counselor acts as consultant to help the client determine a plan and develop steps to implement the plan. In the action stage, the counselor helps the client carry out his plans and continues to support and encourage him to hang in there. The counselor tries to help the client deal with any sense of conflict, or reservations about change with reassurance. When the client reaches the maintenance stage, the counselor reinforces what the client has accomplished and supports the new skills learned.

Comment for the Reader: There can be a couple of pitfalls with motivation that we should talk a little more about. First of all, while treatment is client driven, so to speak, the counselor must have clear ideas about what may be in the client's best interest. While they must understand and respect the client's right to autonomy (making their own decisions), they must also have a guiding sense of direction. That is our responsibility. Treatment needs to be collaborative. It is our job to try to assist the client with motivation, based on the client's own drives, not ours.

In other words, the client may want to continue using drugs. They may also want a fulfilling relationship, or buy a business, or go to school, or be in a band – whatever. Their chances of accomplishing any of those things are greatly improved if the client does not use drugs. So, even though the client has their heels dug in, telling you that they choose to use, and you believe it's in their best interest not to use . . . use their own motives in life (not yours) to inspire motivation in them. The pitfalls are that some will allow the client to continue to use because, well, . . . they "choose to" . . . and the treatment goal belongs to the client. Some will not be clear within themselves what is the right direction.

CONCLUSION

Individual and group counseling skills are at the heart of practical applications and you will, no doubt, develop a style that works for you, and is effective with your clients. Hopefully, this understanding of some fundamental skills is useful here.

Now we move on and start taking a look at treating co-occurring disorders and understanding the conflicts this approach has met with. The unit provides an overview of psychiatric disorders and their treatment.

UNIT 4 Highlights

CH 13: Group Skills

- Early Group Stages/introductions/members finding their niche in the group/checking trust level/what is the tone of the group?/what can I put out there?/what response will I get?/power and control
- Working Stage/cohesion
- Discharge/leaders/separating/reluctance to leave
- Pitfalls in group work/effects of on-going group turn over/relapse/incarceration/drop-out on the group
- Difficult Members/Central Character wants to be center of attention/Pain in the Neck client frequently disrupts groups/Helper is always soothing and rescuing/Nay Sayer negates everything/Psychotic Clients can be distraction in group/all require special handling
- Dealing with silence/resist urge to rescue group until you know why the group is silent
- Cohesion/common purpose/AA members carry over "we" concept

CH 14: Yalom's Curative Factors

- Instillation of hope/Universality/Imparting Information/Altruism/Family group/Social Skills/Imitative behavior/Interpersonal learning/Cohesion/Catharsis/Accepting responsibility

CH 15: Therapist Communication Skills

- Common themes found in all theory/questioning/understanding/solving problems
- Active listening = paying attention/paraphrasing = repeating using different words/reflecting = paraphrasing and including expressed effect/probing = questioning for insight/interpretation = reflecting and providing meaning/summarizing = putting it all together
- Setting tone/providing support/confronting
- Self-disclosure/in who's interest?

CH 16: Stages of Change and Motivational Interviewing

- Precontemplation = not ready or unable to stop/Contemplation = maybe I have a problem/Preparing = thinking about change, but unsure what to do/Action = starting to make changes/Maintenance = continuing to support changes
- Motivational Interviewing/meet clients where they are/kinder, gentler approach/focuses on strengths not problems/uses empathy not authority, control, and power/reflective listening/open-ended questions/affirmations/summarization

STUDY GUIDE

1) Do you prefer individual counseling or group counseling? Why?
2) What type of difficult group member have you experienced?
3) Which of Yalom's Curative Factors in group therapy are most effective in substance abuse counseling? Why is that?
4) Is motivational interviewing a comfortable approach for you? Why? Why not? If not, what is?

5) What is transference? Why do you think it is important?
6) What is counter-transference? Do you think counter-transference can be useful?

References

Andres-Hyman, R. (2004, December). *Recovery Core Values.* Handout Presented at Connecticut Department of Mental Health and Addiction Services Education and Training, Hartford CT.

Cole, B.; & Pargament, K. (1999). Spiritual surrender: A paradoxical path to control. *Integrating spirituality into treatment: Resources for practitioners* (pp. 179-198). Washington, DC US: American Psychological Association. doi:10.1037/10327-009.

Corey, G. (2009). *Theory and practice of counseling and psychotherapy* (8th ed.). Belmont, CA: Brooks/Cole.

Delgado, C. (2007). Sense of Coherence, Spirituality, Stress and Quality of Life in Chronic Illness. *Journal of Nursing Scholarship,* 39(3), 229-34. Retrieved April 18, 2009, from ProQuest Psychology Journals database. (Document ID: 1428124701).

Galanter. M. (2008). Spirituality, Evidence-Based Medicine, and Alcoholics Anonymous. *The American Journal of Psychiatry,* 165(12), 1514-7. Retrieved April 18, 2009, from ProQuest Psychology Journals database. (Document ID: 1607951671).

Henson, B. (2008). Axis I disorders, dual diagnosis, and health-related quality of life: Results from the National Epidemiologic Survey on Alcohol and Related Conditions (NESARC). *Dissertation Abstracts International,* 68, Retrieved from PsycINFO database.

Jacobs, E.E.; Masson, R.L.; & Harvill, R.L. (2009). Group counseling: Strategies and skills. Belmont, CA: Thomson Brooks/Cole.

Koenig, H.G. (2007). *Spirituality in patient care.* Conshohocken, PA: Templeton Press.

Lese, K., & MacNair-Semands, R. (2000). The Therapeutic Factors Inventory: Development of a scale. Group, 24(4), 303-317. doi:10.1023/A:1026616626780.

Liberman, R.P. (2008). Principles and Practice of Psychiatric Rehabilitation: An Empirical Approach. *The American Journal of Psychiatry,* 165(7), 924-925. Retrieved April 18, 2009, from ProQuest Psychology Journals database. (Document ID: 1508355881).

Okun, B.F. (2002). Effective helping: Interviewing and counseling techniques (6th ed.). Pacific Grove, CA: Brooks/Cole.

MacMaster, S.A. (2004). Harm reduction: a new perspective on substance abuse services. [Electronic Version] *Social Work,* 49(3), 356-364.

Narcotics Anonymous. (1984). Van Nuys, CA: World Service Office.

Pargament, K. (1997). The psychology of religion and coping: Theory, research, practice. New York, NY US: Guilford Press. Retrieved from PsycINFO database.

Pargament, K.; Smith, B.; Koenig, H.; & Perez, L. (1998). Patterns of positive and negative religious coping with major life stressors. *Journal for the Scientific Study of Religion,* 37(4), 710-724.

Pray, M., & Watson, L. (2008). Effectiveness of day treatment for dual diagnosis patients with severe chronic mental illness. *Journal of Addictions Nursing,* 19(3), 141-149. doi:10.1080/10884600802306008.

Prochaska, J.O.; Diclemente, C.C.; Norcross, J.C. (1992). In search of how people change: applications to addictive behaviors. [Electronic Version] American Psychologist, 47(9), 1102-1114.

Scherling, D.H. (2004, October). *Hopeful Conversations: Inspiring Recovery Through Motivational Interviewing.* Handout Presented at Connecticut Department of Mental Health and Addiction Services Education and Training, Middletown, CT.

Temple University; Spirituality protects against depression better than church attendance. (2008, November). *Psychology & Psychiatry Journal,* 9. Retrieved April 18, 2009, from ProQuest Psychology Journals database. (Document ID: 1590031151).

Yalom, I.D. & Leszcz, M. (2005). The theory and practice of group psychotherapy. (5th ed.). NY: Basic Books.

UNIT 5/Co-occurring Disorders and Their Treatment

Introduction

Substance abuse addiction is not a new problem. However, more recently Inaba and Cohen (2006) stated that 44% of those treated for alcohol and 64% of those treated for other substances carry another psychiatric diagnosis (other than substance abuse). There are 7-10 million individuals in the U.S. with co-occurring disorders (Prochaski et al., 2005). There is a plethora of research that supports treatment of co-occurring disorders; i.e., anxiety and addiction, depression and addiction, schizophrenia and addiction, and so forth (Inaba & Cohen, 2004; Mojtabai, 2004; Tiet & Mausbach, 2007; Timko, Moos, & Dixon, 2005; McGovern et al., 2007; Granholm et al., 2003; Pray & Watson, 2008). Co-occurring disorders pose confounding problems as the substance abuse problem can exacerbate the mental health disorder and the mental health disorder can exacerbate the substance abuse. Also, while an overwhelming majority of substance abuse clients show up with psychiatric symptoms, sometimes it is necessary to wait up to 8 weeks to get a clear diagnosis that is not substance induced (Fals-Stewart & Lucent, 1994). It is important to distinguish between having symptoms of a psychiatric disorder and having a pre-existing mental illness. It is not unusual for clients to come in with mental illness, the majority of which dissipate in a short while (Inaba & Cohen, 2000). Substance induced mental illness can occur because of drug use or during withdrawal.

Nonetheless, there are many reasons for increased numbers of people with co-occurring disorders: there are fewer mental health hospitals, there is greater substance usage, there are a greater number of professionals today, and there is more knowledge today regarding substance use (Inaba & Cohen, 2000).

Substance-induced disorders can include poor impulse control (violence, suicide, unsafe sex), sleep issues, anxiety and depression, panic, cognitive difficulties, and psychosis. This is true for alcohol, stimulants, cannabis, and opiates (Inaba & Cohen, 2000). It may take weeks or even months for cognitive functions to return to a balanced state. Often people cannot work toward a goal, have a low frustration level, express feelings by their behavior, are in denial, have no hope for the future, fear rejection, test limits, and lie. These are all indications of arrested emotional development presenting with character traits of children (Inaba & Cohen, 2000). People with co-occurring disorders never worked through issues and stresses as adolescents and now avoid difficult emotions (Inaba & Cohen, 2000).

Dual-diagnosed clients face greater obstacles than uni-dimensional diagnoses. Co-occurring disorders exacerbate each other; that is, substance use impacts on other mental health issues and mental health issues impact on substance use (Doweiko, 2009). Dual- diagnosed clients have lower quality of life than those with a single diagnosis (Henson, 2004). Dual-diagnosed clients relapse more frequently (Mehr, 2001). Denial of a sub-stance issue can be greater; noncompliance in treatment is more frequent (Doweiko, 2009).

Also, co-occurring disorders give credence to the notion of individuals self-medicating knowingly or unwittingly; self-medicating in order to cope with their mental health symptoms.

> *Comment for the Reader:* Just remember, co-occurring issues greatly impact on each other and recovery rates and quality of life are poorer for dual-diagnosed individuals, which is why it has become the focus of treatment.

CHAPTER 17

Co-occurring Disorders and Their Treatment

Treatment of co-occurring disorders also presents its own sets of problems. The mental health system does not like to take substance abusers because clients can be disruptive and manipulative in treatment. The substance abuse system does not like to take individuals with mental health disorders because they may be distractible. (Inaba & Cohen, 2000). In other words, clients who are in a mental health program and are continuing to use drugs/alcohol may come to the program high, with alcohol on their breath, or recovering from the effects of drugs/alcohol, such as nodding out in groups. Their attendance may be sporadic and participation minimal. Clients in a substance abuse program who are experiencing mental health symptoms; i.e., depression, anxiety, manic behavior, voices, and so forth, may have a difficult time in group and possibly be a distraction for other members.

Treatment in the past has been sequential, but it has been questionable as to which came first – the mental health problem or the substance abuse problem. Today, more programs are treating both concurrently (Inaba & Cohen, 2000). However, this has been a process wrought with obstacles and controversy because the approaches to mental health treatment and substance abuse treatment have their differences (Inaba & Cohen, 2000). Not only is there disparity between philosophical approaches, but theoretical framework, methods and techniques, different perspectives on collaboration, and different levels of training between the two fields (Inaba & Cohen, 2006). Both camps, however, have the desire to and are moving toward a more holistic approach (Inaba & Cohen, 2006).

Only recently have agencies begun to treat co-occurring disorders simultaneously. For years, clients have been shuffled back and forth between the mental health system and the substance-abuse treatment system. Substance abuse programs had a problem accepting these clients before their mental illness had been treated, because they were "disorganized or disruptive" (Inaba & Cohen, 2004, p.453). Mental health programs were reluctant to take substance abusers because they were "disruptive and manipulative" (Inaba & Cohen, 2004, p. 453). Substance abuse facilities thought if they treated the mental illness, the substance abuse would go away, and mental health providers thought that if they dealt with the substance abuse the mental health problems would resolve themselves. Meanwhile, dual-diagnosed clients' quality of life is adversely affected (Astas et al., 2008; Singh et al., 2005; Bizarri et al., 2005; Welsh et al., 1993; Henson, 2008). The need to address co-occurring disorders is propelling this new dual diagnosis treatment paradigm we have been speaking of.

The American Society of Addiction Medicine (ASAM) has created taxonomy of a dual diagnosis treatment program model. It recognizes three categories of dual diagnosis capable programs: 1) Addiction Services Only (ASO) targeting individuals with primary substance abuse issues and either no or minimal co-occurring problems 2) Dual Diagnosis Capable (DDC) treating those with co-occurring disorders, but who are less severe and more stable 3) Dual Diagnosed Enhanced (DDE) are responsive to those with varying degrees of severity and stability. Programs are encouraged to at least be DDC.

There have been differences in the ways in which the mental health community and the substance abuse community approach treatment of clients. Substance abuse providers have been reluctant to take mentally ill clients because they are too dysfunctional without medication (Inaba & Cohen, 2000). This is mainly because they may just be inattentive (Inaba & Cohen, 2000). A study of a number of dual diagnosed clients at a veterans' hospital demonstrated that the majority was mildly to severely cognitively impaired and that it was difficult for them to participate in treatment (Blume, Davis, & Schmaling, 1999). Finn et al., (1999) also found reduced cognitive functioning in alcoholics with co-morbidity. Medication is often a necessary element of effective integrated treatment to treat the mental illness as well as to facilitate sobriety (Levy & Mann, 1987; Minkoff, 1987; Minkoff, 1989). Mental health providers are reluctant to take substance abusers because they are too disruptive without becoming drug free first (Inaba & Cohen, 2000). There has been avoidance and confusion regarding treating dual diagnosis. Inaba and Cohen (2000) state that treatment of the dual-diagnosed client has historically been sequential or parallel. In other words, mental health treatment and substance abuse treatment would follow one or the other in order. Furthermore, it has always been unclear if the mental health issue preceded the substance abuse issue or vice versa. Both may be true depending upon the individual and their circumstances. Again, mental health professionals have thought that if you treat the underlying psychological problem, the substance abuse will go away. The substance abuse treatment providers have thought that if you help the client become abstinent the psychological problems will become manageable, minimize, or go away altogether. While there is truth to both statements, providers are beginning to realize that one-third to three-fourths of their clients have co-occurring disorders and that concurrent treatment is necessary.

At times, treatment would be concurrent with two different providers. Treatment facilities are now beginning to address dual diagnosis simultaneously. While there is still disparity and controversy in practice between the mental health and substance abuse camps, both are working toward a closer, compatible, and more complementary relationship.

However, there are some complications to work out. Mental health providers are more accepting of a partial remission or recovery from the problem, whereas substance abuse providers aim for lifelong abstinence. As discussed, there is today a renewed interest and pursuit of a harm reduction paradigm (MacMaster, 2002). Remember that harm reduction embraces goals of reduced (drug) usage, reduced frequency and/or quantity of drugs used, and reduced crises and consequences as a result of alcohol and other drug usage. Next, clients may be more reticent to seek help through the mental health system than from drug and alcohol treatment programs, due to the stigma related to psychiatric illness (Inaba & Cohen, 2000). Of course, the reverse can be true as well, but frequently clients and their families believe one can more readily recover from addiction than mental illness chronic, severe, and prolonged problems. Another issue providing controversy is that mental health providers frequently rely on medication to treat clients. The substance abuse camp is divided between an approach of complete abstinence and a harm reduction approach, such as methadone programs (Inaba & Cohen, 2000). Old timers in AA will balk at newcomers' usage of medications, which does not help this dilemma for the client, because they are receiving a double message. While the medications may help them feel better, sleep better – they may feel their recovery is limited. There can also be a dichotomy (a two-way split) of provider approach. Mental health treatment often relies on case management to guide the client through whatever services may seem necessary, where as substance abuse treatment usually places this responsibility on the client because they do not want to enable the client (Inaba & Cohen, 2000). However, there is also a trend toward providing the client with holistic services, and as a result case management, in some cases, is blended in with substance abuse treatment.

Inaba and Cohen (2000) suggest that treatment approaches for mental health clients, substance abuse clients and dual-diagnosed clients currently presents a conundrum of perspectives. Current psychotherapeutic approaches are often supportive with an emphasis on the therapeutic alliance or relationship; i.e., humanistic psychology. While these things are not unimportant in substance abuse programs, treatment programs often continue to use confrontation methods with the client. And, there are certainly times when it is necessary to break through the denial that accompanies substance abuse issues. Mental health practitioners may find confrontation approaches inappropriate and this can be a very real dilemma when a client is not responding to substance abuse treatment due to a mental illness. It then becomes difficult to apply the same behavioral expectations found in program policy to dual-diagnosed clients. In terms of confrontation as a treatment technique in substance abuse programs, motivational interviewing (MI) methods utilizing Prochaski and DiClemente's (1994) *stages of change* is now widely supported as a preferred approach. MI is a gentler, subtler means of eliciting response from clients and is more collaborative than directive. It recognizes that clients are going to be in various stages of a continuum involving a pre-contemplative stage, contemplation of the recognition of a problem, preparing to deal with the problem, and then actually taking action regarding the problem. MI and the stages of change recognize that recovery is a process and that confronting a client who is precontemplative, that is, either has not begun to think about whether they have a problem or simply do not think they have a problem, is not only ineffective but may be harmful by pushing the client away (Miller & Rollnick, 1991).

Another disparity between the mental health and substance abuse fields is that the mental health community is more accustomed to sharing information and collaborating with other providers (Inaba & Cohen, 2000). The mental health field has always consisted of professionally credentialed individuals, whereas in the past, substance abuse counselors have often been recovering persons themselves. It has only been recently that most states are requiring specialized training, certification, licensing and the requirement of continued education. Also, dual diagnosis is being considered its own specialty as opposed to mental health training and substance abuse training singly. Along the same lines, mental health treatment has relied on the scientific method defining best practices. Substance abuse treatment approach, which has been based on Alcoholics Anonymous philosophy, tradition, and personal experiences of counselors, is no longer sufficient. Current best practices include the disease model (the basis for AA) as one of several approaches, not the sole approach. The mental health community on the other hand has much to learn from the substance abuse community, particularly with regard to self-experiences and spirituality in recovery (Inaba & Cohen, 2000).

Another philosophical difference in a mental health approach vs. a substance abuse approach is that mental health practices are unmistakably aimed at preventing the client from getting worse (Inaba & Cohen, 2000). Substance abuse practice, borrowing from a 12-step (AA) approach believes that an individual needs to hit bottom before being able to be receptive to recovery; that this is what it takes to break through the denial that accompanies addiction (Inaba & Cohen, 2000). While this thinking has become outdated with the advent of MI, which can help the client recognize their problem, it is still believed to be true by many and adds to misconception in treatment.

Mental health treatment has always been individualized, whereas AA philosophy has been the basis for almost all substance abuse programs in the past, and it was believed to be the only successful method of treatment. In reality, both approaches need to be integrated when treating the dual-diagnosed client, including a motivational approach, cognitive behavioral methods, and AA (Inaba & Cohen, 2000).

There is one more aspect of dual-diagnosis treatment that remains problematic and it lies in the inherent difficulty of proper diagnosis (Inaba & Cohen, 2000). Mental health practitioners may misdiagnose clients in early treatment with mental illness, as opposed to substance-induced mental illness, and the reverse is true as well. Substance abuse professionals may miss diagnosing mental illness, believing symptoms are substance induced. Dual-diagnosis treatments sometimes now take a wait and see approach before diagnosing and medicating. There is much confusion and multiple conflicting approaches that still exist in the field. As a result, a client may have to insufferably wait to be medicated in one program, versus another client who may be inappropriately medicated in another (Inaba & Cohen, 2000).

Despite all the controversy previously described, one thing is emerging that is clear and virtually undisputed: clients do not have the option of separating their mental illness from their substance abuse, so why should treatment programs? (Osher, 2001). In other words, the clients' needs are clear; they require treatment for co-morbid disorders and treatment programs should follow suit. Research supports the theory that clients with co-occurring disorders need to be treated simultaneously for both disorders in the same program (Kosten & Ziedonis, 1997). In the event that this is not possible, treatment needs to be collaboratively concurrent with linked agencies (Kosten & Ziedonis, 1997).

Furthermore, this is another reason for the paradigm shift from needs-based therapy to strengths-based perspectives or person-centered therapy. Both mental health and substance abuse practitioners have historically viewed clients based on their needs or deficits, which was founded in traditional psychodynamic psychology. As the prevailing school of thought has shifted to a humanistic, existential direction, there has been an increased effort to base treatment on a client's strengths which form the basis of integrated dual diagnosis treatment (IDDT). According to the CT Department of Mental Health and Addiction Services (DMHAS) which has adopted the national Substance Abuse and Mental Health Administration's (SAMHSA) proposed model of recovery and recovery-oriented services, IDDT consists of several basic recovery premises.

These premises have filtered down from SAMHSA to the state and community level. State agencies and government-funded private non-profit agencies will subscribe to them. In Connecticut, the Department of Mental Health and Addiction Services (DMHAS) provides this material, which is contained in the following discussion. First, all clients are individual and have specific needs, objectives, attitudes, behaviors, and expectations for recovery. Clients, whether being treated for mental health issues, substance abuse, or both, have things in common; however, the directions and pursuits that people choose may be different. Clients are encouraged to actively participate in their treatment and recovery process. Treatment must be approached holistically. Clients must be able to collaborate in every determining phase of their treatment plan. Nomenclature will reflect individualized recovery-based language; i.e., "Recovery Plans" shall replace "Treatment Plans." This strengths-based approach shall be used and promoted. There should not be any "wrong doors" when entering treatment service. A client's choice must be respected in all matters. Programming must be flexible to incorporate individual recovery plans.

IDDT has determined that there are several Recovery Dimensions. They include understanding how behaviors effect recovery; hope, confidence and commitment; understanding and accepting oneself; relationships with family, friends, and supportive others; maintaining recovery; supports in the community to enhance recovery; promoting recovery; and becoming an empowered citizen. The need to address co-occurring disorders is propelling a new dual-diagnosis treatment paradigm. It is estimated that 10 million Americans suffer from co-occurring disorders (Mojtabai, 2004). As touched on previously, The American Society of Addiction Medicine (ASAM) has created taxonomy of a dual-diagnosis treatment program model. It recognizes three categories of dual-diagnosis capable programs: Addiction Services Only (ASO); Dual Diagnosis Capable (DDC); and Dual Diagnosed Enhanced (DDE). Programs are encouraged to at least be DDC. Most are ASO due to financial and staffing restriction. Few are DDE due to costs and policy prohibitions (McGovern et al., 2007). ASAM is providing a roadmap to DDC programs that would include a program structure that contains a mission, structure and financing, and a format for the delivery of services. It must also have a program milieu addressing the physical, social, and cultural environment. It must be capable of clinical process, including assessment (entry into services, screening, and diagnosis) and treatment (pharmacological and psychosocial best practices). It must provide continuity of care for both substance use and psychiatric needs and have appropriate staffing certified, licensed, and trained in co-occurring disorders (McGovern et al., 2007; McGovern et al., 2007). Federal, state, and local government owned or funded facilities are more likely to service dual-diagnosed clients (Mojabai, 2004). A large number of agencies catering to clients with co-occurring disorders do not yet offer full services (Mojabai, 2004).

There are difficulties setting up dual-diagnosed programs; substance abuse recovery and mental illness recovery have often sent conflicting messages to the client in the past (Timko, Dixon, & Moos, 2005). However, increased need for dual-diagnosed services has heightened the pressure for agencies to become full service and yield better outcomes for their clients than parallel or sequential treatment (Timko, Dixon, & Moos, 2005).

Tiet and Mausbach (2007), in a literature review, state that best practices with psychiatric symptoms and substance abuse are effective with dual-diagnosed clients. However, efficacy with an integrated model is uncertain at this time. McGovern et al., (2007) concur that there have been insufficient objective studies with the ASAM model as well. Nonetheless, in an earlier pilot study, dual-diagnosed treatment was found to reduce the number of psychiatric inpatient hospitalizations by 60% (Granholm et al., 2003).

Clients with dual-diagnosed needs often have exacerbating circumstances, such as homelessness, a history of violence, a history of incarceration, and non-compliance with treatment and medication. Treatment outcomes are typically worse than for clients with substance abuse issues alone (Pray & Watson, 2008). Pray and Watson (2008) did examine clinical outcomes in a dual-diagnosis day program. The study demonstrated the longer clients remained in the program, the higher the remission rate. Also, those with a year abstinence were less likely to relapse.

Paralleling the shift from one-dimensional treatment to integrated treatment, the criminal justice system is following suit. Smith (1999), in a literature review, state that pilot integrated programs reflect lower criminal justice costs, increased productivity and higher functioning in clients, less cost to the taxpayer, and a decrease in recidivism.

Dual diagnosis quality of life. Dual-diagnosed clients' quality of life is adversely affected as a result of their co-morbid disorder (Astas et al., 2008; Singh et al., 2005; Bizarri et al., 2005; Welsh et al., 1993; Henson, 2008). Magura et al., (2007) utilized this assumption when studying the effects of concurrent treatment in this program evaluation. This study only reviews the outcome of one dual-focus program. While it may not be sufficient to apply to all dual-focus programs, it points in a direction; i.e., dual diagnosed persons left untreated face a poor quality of life.

Drake (2006) studied the long-term course of clients with schizophrenia and substance abuse disorders over 10 years. Participants improved steadily over 10 years in the outcome domains of symptoms, substance abuse, institutionalization, functional status, and quality of life. The quantitative study exemplifies the poor quality of life and unique obstacles faced by dual-diagnosed clients. One major limitation of this study is that mental health recovery is difficult to define and measure.

McNeil, Binder, and Robinson (2005) correlated incarceration and homelessness with dual diagnosis. Dual-diagnosed persons represented a substantial number of homeless that had been jailed. The study inadvertently suggested that the Correctional System is assuming responsibility for this dual-diagnosed population. This study was done in San Francisco; it is possible that rates of incarcerated dual-diagnosed persons are higher than other parts of the country. However, it is likely that many urban areas face similar situations.

Probably most profound but not surprising, research involving a cross-sectional assessment of substance use clients, psychiatric clients, and dual-diagnosed clients, dual diagnosed clients' quality of life scores were significantly lower than the other groups (Henson, 2008).

> *Comment for the Reader:* It may be surprising to many . . . it was to me . . . that there is so much conflict between the mental health model for treatment and the substance model for treatment. Brother/sister facilities become at odds with each other over who should take which client. Go figure. It's hard to believe that a rift has developed between the two. I mean, why can't we all just get along, right? Well, it's the merging of two different worlds of orientation, so I guess difficulty is going to be inherent. The good news is that most agree that substance abuse and mental health issues need to be treated simultaneously.

CHAPTER 18

DSM-IV-TR

The Diagnostic Statistical Manual-IV-TR (DSM) is a major diagnostic tool for the assessment of psychiatric disorders. Despite being the subject of much controversy, it is a standard in the field. The DSM represents a huge undertaking and a team effort of over 1,000 contributors answering to a task force. Its credibility and utility extend to clinical, research, and educational purposes supported by extensive empirical findings (American Psychiatric Association, 2004). The term mental disorder is used to describe "clinically significant behavior or psychological syndrome or pattern that occurs in an individual associated with distress, disability, or loss of freedom." The DSM is used clinically, educationally, and in research settings by individuals with clinical training and experience, and is not meant to be applied mechanically. It is meant to present guidelines to assist clinical judgment . . . "not a cookbook." A diagnosis may be justified even if it doesn't meet full criteria, given the intensity and severity of symptoms. Lack of experience with DSM will reduce its utility (American Psychiatric Association, 2004).

DSM usage can be part of a comprehensive evaluation and the first part of a treatment plan along with significant additional factors and information. DSM reflects a "consensus of current information," but not to be applied in all situations. Its purpose is to provide a clear description in order to diagnose, discuss, research, and treat (American Psychiatric Association, 2004).

The DSM makes use of the ICD classification of codes. It is found in various places in DSM. It is fundamental to record keeping when dealing with insurance companies and government agencies. There is a 5th digit of the code that designates subtypes (i.e., delusional or grandiose when discussing psychosis) and specifiers for increased specificity (i.e., depression with melancholic features). Severity is described in seven ways:

1) mild: few symptoms
2) moderate: functional impairment
3) severe: in excess of diagnosis
4) in partial remission: only one symptom remains;
5) in full remission: no symptoms left, but it is still relevant
6) prior history or reoccurrence: when full criteria is not met or it is a new episode
7) provisional: when there is a presumption that criteria will be met (American Psychiatric Association, 2004).

The main diagnosis, listed first, is the client's reason for the visit. If it is inpatient it is the chief complaint that may be ambiguous; i.e., in a case of dual diagnosis. Multiple diagnoses can be listed along with the multi-axial (categories) description (American Psychiatric Association, 2004). Axis I refers to the chief complaint; maybe substance abuse, mental health, or both. Axis II refers to personality disorders. Axis III refers to general medical conditions. Axis IV refers to psychosocial and environmental problems. Axis V is a global assessment score (GAF) which is based on the severity of dysfunction.

The phrase 'not otherwise specified' (NOS) is used when symptoms are in the same classification, but do not meet specific features, when symptoms are not included in the classification, when there is uncertainty of cause, or when there is incomplete data. There are also other ways of representing an uncertain diagnosis (American Psychiatric Association, 2004).

At other times, there may not be sufficient information about a client to meet diagnostic criteria, but the counselor is leaning toward a particular diagnosis. The diagnosis may used but specified as 'provisional.' This means that the client will most likely fall into this diagnosis once all criteria have been established.

There are times when the clinician is exploring certain possibilities and may use a diagnosis and specify it as 'rule out.' This means the client's symptoms 'look like' this diagnosis here, and we are looking for it, but it may not be the case. For example, a client may come into a drug program referred by family services. Family services suspects an alcohol problem and sends the client in for an evaluation. Perhaps the client's self-reported history does not support a diagnosis. The clinician may use a 'rule out' in order to observe the client for a potential problem.

DSM is organized into 16 major classifications. Also, it contains "decision trees" which assist in diagnosing by a series of – "if not this, then . . ." DSM diagnostic classifications are:

1) First evident in childhood
2) Delirium, dementia, and other cognitive disorders
3) Mental disorders due to a general medical condition
4) Substance-related disorders
5) Mood disorders
6) Anxiety disorders
7) Somatoform disorders
8) Factitious disorders
9) Dissociative disorders
10) Sexual and gender-identity disorders
11) Eating disorders
12) Sleep disorders

13) Personality disorders

14) Other conditions

Martin et al., (2007) present problems with DSM with regard to substance abuse diagnosis and offer perspective changes to DSM-V. This study shall be exemplified here as it is reflective of the types of presentation of research implying lack of reliability and validity in DSM, as well as presenting recommendations for DSM-V. Criticism for DSM-IV include current substance diagnosis does not have a clear operational definition; there are divergent meanings. Current DSM usage makes for difficulty determining severity due to variation of individual criteria. There is a reported insignificant distinction between abuse and dependence categories. Current definition of tolerance can be applied to the abuse category while it is a dependence criteria. Abuse and dependence are marked by maladaptive behaviors, but actual patterns are not described in DSM. Currently 2 out of 8 criteria for withdrawal produce false positives in community samples. Research supports that there is cannabis withdrawal, but it is not reflected in DSM criteria. "Larger, longer symptoms" can create a false positive diagnosis in dependence criteria despite lack of compulsive usage. Quitting and cutting down is considered evidence of 'repeated efforts to stop' despite cutting down construct may indicate a less severe problem. Continued use in hazardous situations and legal problems may demonstrate inaccurate severity of diagnosis, and may also discriminate against cultural differences and gender bias. The DSM tends to 'pigeon-hole' moderate levels of substance usage into existing categories of diagnosis and is equally less accurate diagnosing more severe levels of use. DSM is largely categorical and does not sufficiently take into account dimensional factors. (In other words, instead of looking at categories of abuse and dependency, look at the level of distress and dysfunction). Lastly, the DSM does not take into account the current commonality of certain co-occurring disorders.

Martin et al., (2007) proposed changes which included dropping the abuse category altogether and illustrated substance dependence on a consumption scale. Define substance dependence based on evidence on a uni-dimensional continuum for substance use problems. Avoid low levels of standards to raise the validity of individual criteria. Change the operational definition of 'tolerance' to include a minimum level of use. The new DSM should utilize consumption scales; i.e., so many drinks in a 2-hour time period 1x weekly. Utilize withdrawal as a physiological feature constituting dependence criteria. Cannabis withdrawal should become part of DSM criteria and further research is required to define features. DSM should clarify that using more and longer occurs due to compulsivity not due to social factors. Separate cutting down and quitting attempts into separate criteria. Illicit substance abuse behavior should be removed as diagnostic criteria for substance dependence, but added to criteria for anti-social disorders. Include criteria for measuring mild to severe categories based on consumption and craving. Consideration should be given to using dimensional scales indicating the severity of usage and describing these features. Group substance use disorders with compulsive disorders and anti-social personality disorders.

> *Comment for the Reader:* Contrary to popular belief, I like the DSM and I like using diagnoses. While a label may be stigmatic, it provides many with a hook to hang their hat. Many suffer through a barrage of symptoms for years and believe that they are just a failure. It can help people to say, "Aha! so THAT's it . . . so this is what's going on with me . . . and that's what it's called . . . there's even a name for it . . . and I'm not the only one who's like this!"

Entry level counselors are typically not going to make mental health diagnoses, but they may report it 'by history.' In other words, if a client reports he has been diagnosed with depression, it may be listed. The entry level counselor may well be making substance abuse diagnoses on an Axis I, particularly if they are doing intake/evaluations. Below is what typical diagnostic impressions may look like:

Axis I	311.00	Depressive Disorder by history
	304.20	Cocaine Dependence
Axis II	V71.09	Deferred
Axis III	492.80	Emphysema
Axis IV		Family problems, unemployment
Axis V	45	Highest in past year 50

CHAPTER 19

SUBSTANCE ABUSE VS. SUBSTANCE DEPENDENCE

Despite current criticisms of the DSM, it is widely used by insurance companies and thus treatment facilities alike assisting in determining the right level of care for your client. The insurance companies have set up criteria for different levels of care and depending on the diagnosis you have arrived at, you may have to justify why your client needs a particular level of care.

The hallmark distinctions between chemical abuse and chemical dependency are two factors of substance usage – tolerance and withdrawal. Tolerance is defined as needed to use more of a substance to achieve the same effect. Withdrawal refers to physiological changes the body undergoes when the particular drug leaves the system, causing distress and impairment. DSM lists withdrawal symptoms for each drug separately under that drug category. The client will not fall into a dependence category if they do not experience tolerance or withdrawal. Substance abuse drug listings in DSM include alcohol, cocaine, opiates, cannabis, amphetamines, hallucinogens, and inhalants.

Criteria for substance dependence include three or more of the following in a 12-month period (APA, 2004).

(1) Tolerance

(2) Withdrawal

(3) Taking the substance in larger quantity over a longer period of time than intended

(4) There is a persistent desire for unsuccessful efforts to cut down or control usage

(5) A great deal of time is spent obtaining, using, or recovering from the effects of substance usage

(6) Important social, occupational, or recreational activities are given up or reduced because of substance use

(7) Continued usage despite knowledge of persistent or recurrent physical or psychological problems most likely caused by the substance

Criteria for substance abuse include:

[A] one of the following over a 12-month period.

(1) Continued use despite failure to meet major role obligations at work, school, or home.

(2) Continued use in physically hazardous situations (like driving)

(3) Recurrent usage despite persistent or recurring social or interpersonal problems caused or made worse by substance usage

[B] The symptoms have never met criteria for dependency

Treatment

Currently, substance abuse treatment is a blend of cognitive behavioral therapy, motivational interviewing (see Chapter 15), and AA philosophy (see Chapters 10, 11, and 24). There are many references to solutions-focused therapy throughout the book, which are essentially CBT skills. The Matrix System exemplifies one solutions-focused effort described below (Ramson et al., 2004).

CBT in substance abuse treatment involves a structured effort to help clients stop using, and provide basic early recovery tools and specific relapse prevention skills. There are two central objectives: first, change is possible and second, the skills presented are best combined with self-help and spiritual supports in the community. Tools center around an understanding of triggers – internal and external, and learning to modulate them. A 12-step introduction is provided, and biological issues and other common difficulties in early recovery are provided. Relapse-prevention groups are oriented around pitfalls in recovery, such as boredom, work issues, the impact of guilt and shame, staying busy, maintaining motivation, remaining honest, complete abstinence, complacency, sex, trust, spirituality, managing money, self-care, dangerous emotions, managing stress and anger, friends and relationships, and 12-step philosophies.

Another example of a CBT approach to mental health recovery is Pathways to Recovery (Ridgway et al., 2002). I believe it is equally as effective for substance abusers. It is a strengths-based approach facilitating identification of personal strengths. It is aimed at helping individuals find empowerment within them. The exercises take on a strong spiritual flavor, utilizing hope and courage as a foundation along with bolstering attitudes, behavior, motivation, and responsibility. The exercises guide the individual through developing direction in their recovery as well as maneuvering obstacles, staying focused, and developing spiritually. It includes sections on relationships and friendships, relaxation techniques, maintaining balance in recovery, and supports the benefits of storytelling.

Comment for the Reader: I've mentioned a couple of times that people come into treatment for different reasons and at various stages of drug use, abuse, and dependency, and thus with varying degrees of motivation. There are many times when this is a problem in the treatment group. As you can imagine, those who are not serious about it can contaminate others, and often those who are serious get upset with those who are not because they feel it impedes their progress in treatment. And they're right! This is just a reality of treatment programs; it goes with the territory.

We need to remember a few things. 1) if someone doesn't want it (recovery), there is nothing that you can say right. And 2) if someone does want it, you won't be able to say anything wrong. 3) People in programs know who's serious and who's not, and those serious about it should be encouraged to hang out with the other winners. 4) These things need to be addressed in groups on a regular basis because it comes up often. The fact that recovery is a process can be raised; those who now want recovery can be reminded of a time probably not so long ago that there were not motivated either. Those who are not yet motivated feel some heat to at least look at what's put them there in the first place, and that is all part of the process.

Also, within the text, terms are used interchangeably; i.e., addiction/alcoholism, addict, alcoholic, chemical dependency, and so forth. Let me be clear. Alcohol is, of course, a drug. But the distinction between alcohol and other drugs is a historic one. We have grown accustomed to talking about "drugs and alcohol" when it is all really the same. Alcohol was first recognized as a problem that required treatment. Other drugs followed suit. Also, there is the legal distinction. Alcohol is legal, but most other drugs are not. But, we should all be clear that when discussing addiction, there is no distinction – legal, moral, historic, or otherwise.

CHAPTER 20

Psychiatric Disorders

In this section, I have categorized psychiatric disorders in three areas: neuroses, psychoses, and personality disorders. It is my experience that this basic breakdown is most useful for the beginner counselor. We shall deal with the basics here and with the more common scenarios. My aim is to highlight the key information useful to identifying and treating co-occurring disorders. At this stage, most of you probably won't be the one doing the diagnosing; therefore, the emphasis will be on briefly describing disorders and then providing many best practices in the treatment of these issues. First, to distinguish between neuroses and psychoses; both are classifications of mental functioning. Both involve distress and dysfunctional behavior; however, psychoses involve delusions and/or hallucinations. Delusions are fixed beliefs that are not based in reality. Hallucinations, simply, are when people hear (auditory) and/or see (visual) things that others do not.

Anxiety Disorder

Anxiety is certainly going to be the most prevalent type of neurosis that we see with co-occurring disorders. Well, you say, everyone has anxiety, why is this important? Clinical anxiety is going to be more frequent, more intense, more enduring, and interferes with daily functioning (Tafrate, 2006). There are different types of anxiety disorders. Their basic descriptions are as the DSM-IV describes them (APA, 2004).

Generalized anxiety disorder (GAD) is associated with excessive worry and physical symptoms such as rapid breathing, perspiring, chest pains, trembling, palpitations, and so forth, as well as a fear of dying or losing control. This must continue for six months or more to meet criteria for a GAD diagnosis (APA, 2004).

Post-traumatic stress disorder (PTSD) is described as re-experiencing a traumatic event along with increased stress and an avoidance of triggers that may be associated with the event; i.e., sexual assault or war experiences (APA, 2004).

Panic disorders are reoccurring unexpected attacks of anxiety/panic that generate much concern. Symptoms are similar to those described above regarding GAD. There exists a panic cycle involving increased focus on a stimulus, reoccurring physical symptoms as described, negative thoughts about the stimulus and the physical symptoms, and then increased symptoms. This cycle may be accompanied with feelings of unreality; times takes on a new dimension, senses become acute, and greater sensitivity to surroundings is enhanced (APA, 2004).

Agoraphobia is an avoidance of places or situations where it may be difficult to escape from; i.e., while driving, taking public transportation, waiting in line, crowds, stores, restaurants, open spaces, being home alone, elevators, and so forth (APA, 2004).

Obsessive-compulsive disorders: obsession is associated with reoccurring thoughts, pictures, and distressing impulses; and compulsions are associated with repetitive behaviors that people feel driven to in response to their obsessive thinking (APA, 2004). People may be washers, checkers, repeaters, excessive order, hoarders, thinkers, ritualizers, ruminators, and avoiders (Tafrate, 2004). Shame can be an obsession. Actions are compulsive.

Social anxiety occurs when a person experiences significant anxiety in situations where they feel like they are being evaluated, which often leads to avoiding those situations (APA, 2004).

TREATMENT FOR ANXIETY DISORDER

There are various techniques for handling anxiety of different kinds. Clients often find it useful to track their daily anxiety or panic attacks (Tafrate, 2004). This helps to gauge what they are experiencing and compare with previous experiences that they have gotten themselves through. One can keep a daily mood record scaled from one to eight measuring anticipation, worry, and panic, and keep track of average anxiety and/or depression. A panic attack record kept with date, time, duration; did it occur alone, with a friend, with a stranger, with family, and the symptoms. Self-monitoring in these ways helps the client become more familiar with the process and the knowledge that it will pass. The client can learn physical control to aid with their symptoms (Tatrate, 2004). Deep breathing, inhaling slowly to the count of seven and exhaling slowly to the count of seven can offset the rapid, short breathing that accompanies panic. Closing ones eyes and visualizing relaxing powers coming into each and every part of their body can offset the tightness and tenseness that is experienced. This is a slow and methodical process relaxing one part of the body at a time. Sometimes, the proper medication regimen is necessary, appropriate, and useful. Another helpful method with anxiety is cognitive restructuring (Tatrate, 2004). Most people with anxiety overestimate the likelihood of the worst-case scenario. While anything is possible, and you can say that to the client, have them actually estimate, how likely is it that _______ occurs? From 0 to 100%, what is the probability of ________ happening? Help the client reach a realistic estimate of probability and then spell it out for them. So, there is only a 5% chance of this occurring; that means there is a 95% chance that it will not happen. Also, people tend to think in catastrophic terms; that they would never be able to handle a particular situation. It can be helpful to play it out . . . well, if that did happen, this is what I'd do. Have the client be specific about the worst of their fear; i.e., "I'll die," or "I'll go out of control." Anxiety clients see the world as a dangerous place and worrying protects them. Exposure to the object of anxiety can be helpful. Just like the child who is afraid of the water is encouraged to put just their big toe in first; just the toe, and go on from there.

For people with dual diagnosis, PTSD is a fairly common co-occurrence. Sometimes clients are reluctant to talk about the issue, but it is important for clients to know they are not alone. 30-59% of women and 11-38% of men in treatment have current PTSD (Najavits, 2002). It is likely, thus, that more than one person in your group will be experiencing PTSD. PTSD clients use substances for a variety of reasons; to escape from re-occurring thoughts or feelings, to ease the pain, and to cope through the day (Tafrate, 2004). There are two central themes with PTSD (Tafrate, 2004); one is secrecy. People are often ashamed and want to keep people from knowing. The second theme is control in this regard. People with PTSD typically have had something occur over which they had no control. They have lost control over their substance use as well. Healing is often about honesty and gaining control. PTSD and substance abuse increase the likelihood of the other; recovery is about keeping oneself safe from further trauma or substance abuse. Using substances can increase or decrease PTSD symptoms (Tafrate, 2004). So can abstinence. It is important for the client to know what patterns exist for them to cope better with the recovery process (Tafrate, 2004).

Grounding is a method of regaining focus when trauma emotions are resurfacing and one is overwhelmed with pain (Najavits, 2002). Najavits (2002) explains the processes. It is a way of detaching and can be done anywhere and anytime and no one has to know. It is used when faced with a trigger, rage, craving, or whenever emotional pain goes beyond a 6 (0-10: 10 is extreme). Keep your eyes open, scan the room, and turn the light on; all to stay in touch with the present. Do not talk or write about the feelings – the goal is to distract from the negative emotions, not focus on them. Stay neutral; avoid 'good' or 'bad' statements about things; instead, focus on physical qualities of the room. The ceiling is low, the walls are blue, not whether you like that or not. Focus on the present not the past or future. Grounding is not the same as relaxation techniques; it is more active, focused on relieving negative emotions, and is a distraction strategy. There are three ways to ground: mental, physical, and soothing. Mental refers to focusing on your thinking. Physical means focusing on your senses. Soothing is talking to yourself in a very loving and kind way.

Mental grounding can include describing your surroundings in detail; playing category games (what are types of dogs?); describing an everyday activity in great detail (baking a pie); imagining (changing your TV channel, skating away from the pain); reading something out loud. Physical grounding can include running cool or warm water over your hands; holding your chair tightly; digging your heals into the floor; keeping a special object with you (a stone, ring, token) that you can hold; jumping up and down; noticing your body (wiggling your toes in your socks, feeling the back of the chair); stretching; clenching and releasing your fists; walking slowly (noticing each footstep, stating left, right . . .); eating something and describing the flavors to yourself. Soothing grounding can include talking to yourself like you might a small child (support and encourage yourself); thinking of favorite things (people, places, things); remembering an inspiring song; picturing a safe place; giving yourself coping statements (I can do this . . .). Grounding works and may take practice. Practice often; practice doing it faster; practice doing it slowly (20 min.); see what works best; develop your own techniques; start when you have an early sign of a trigger; write down methods on an index card to have with you when you need it.

Comment for the Reader: In recovery, they talk about having a "toolbox." And our objective is to supply our clients with as many tools as possible. It's good to try and get familiar with as many techniques as possible.

Depressive Disorders

Depressive disorders are also known as Mood Disorders. Depression can go hand in hand with anxiety and is also a common co-occurring disorder. A word of caution about all co-occurring diagnoses: be sure you are not looking at physiological effects of a substance or post-acute withdrawal syndrome. Both can look the same. Doctors will rarely diagnose or medicate before they have an opportunity to see what the client looks like clean. An exception to that may be when a client has an established history of a diagnosis and perhaps has gone off their medications.

We usually know what depression looks like, so let's look at symptoms of depression first. The DSM-IV describes them as follows: Affective (emotional) symptoms include sadness, crying, brooding, anxiety, irritability, paranoia, dysphoria (unpleasant mood), anhedonia (an inability to experience pleasure). Cognitive symptoms include disturbances in one's self-perception, the world, and the future. This can cause social withdrawal, low self-esteem, excessive fears, self-criticism, being critical of others, passiveness, delusions or hallucinations. The individual may have guilt over the past, have a sense of unworthiness in the present; and hopelessness about the future. The individual may be vegetative. Often, symptoms are worse in the morning and improve during the day. These may include sleep issues, like difficulty sleeping or sleeping too much (insomnia and hypersomnia), fatigue, decreased libido, increased or decreased appetite and weight change, difficulty concentrating, and constipation. Other symptoms include anxiety; a preoccupation with death; i.e., wishing one was dead; and planning and/or attempting suicide. Some present with back and neck pain, headaches, stomach pain, and increased awareness of pain.

There are many types of depression; we will focus on the most predominant – major depression, bipolar (manic-depressive) disorder, and dysthymic disorder. According to the DSM-IV, major depression is an extreme or prolonged period of sadness accompanied by a loss of interest or pleasure in life. Bipolar disorder is a sequential episode of mania (a high) and depression (a low). Dysthymic disorder is a continuous moderate level of depression and anxiety.

Major Depression. Everyone gets 'blue' or sad or moody, but major depression is persistent and significantly disrupts an individual's thoughts, feelings, moods, and behavior. It affects women more than men, can occur at any age, and affects all races, ethnic groups, and socio-economic groups. Depression is caused by psychological, biological and environmental factors and is considered a biological brain disorder (Schering, 2006).

There are several chemical neuro-transmitters (messengers) in the brain; particularly relevant to depression are norepinephrine, serotonin, and dopamine. They send electrical signals between brain cells. If there is a chemical imbalance in these transmitters, depression may result. Antidepressants work by increasing the availability of transmitters or by changing the sensitivity of the receptors for these chemical messages (Emmerling, 2008).

As a result of the chemical imbalance described above, there is automatic thinking that arises in response to the self, the world, experiences, and the future. These include sadness; guilt or shame; anger, irritation, annoyance, or resentment; anxiety, worry, fear, nervousness, or panic; inferiority or inadequacy; loneliness; hopelessness or discouragement (Scherling, 2006).

People suffering from depression often develop distorted ways of thinking. These include all-or-nothing thinking; overgeneralization; mental filtering toward negativity and discounting the positive; jumping to conclusions, mind reading, fortune telling (all negative); magnification; emotional reasoning reflecting negative mindset; "should" statements; labeling; and personalization and self-blame (Scherling, 2006).

There are perceptions and attitudes that prevent the individual from listening accurately. These include preoccupation with proving a point; overwhelming belief the other is to blame; a need to be a victim and feel sorry for self; inability to see one's role in the problem; defensive fear of criticism; need to win; entitlement; selfishness; mistrust; fear of conflict; belief that one must be emotionally perfect and not vulnerable in any way; fear of disapproval and rejection; passive aggressiveness (not directly dealing with feelings); hopelessness; low self-esteem; and martyrdom – another type of being a victim (Scherling, 2006).

Treatment for Depressive Disorders

Psychotherapy has proven successful with mild to moderate depression. More severe depression responds well to a combination of medication and counseling.

Harry Stack Sullivan was versed in psychodynamics, but strongly influenced by social psychology. He believed that interpersonal relationships trigger the most significant emotional reactions in people, and developed Interpersonal Therapy (IPT). IPT work with depression focuses on identifying and correcting weak social skills. It aims to resolve exacerbated loss and grief, unresolved disputes, role transitions, and interpersonal deficiencies. IPT relies on the therapeutic relationship as a basis to provide encouragement, communication analysis, and clarification.

Cognitive Behavioral Therapy focuses on identifying and correcting faulty thinking (cognitive distortions as described). It aims to teach identifying skills and corrective strategies when evaluating events or circumstances to avoid inaccurate interpretations. CBT explores thought content and style by investigative questioning and assigning tasks to be practiced. CBT makes use of rewarding successful behaviors and employs relaxation skills, assertiveness training, role-playing, and modeling (Scherling, 2006).

In addition, there are various methods of treating depression. These include providing information about depression, self-help books, reframing perspectives, anxiety management (relaxation, meditation), physical exercise, teaching affirmation skills, teaching coping skills, suicide assessment, sleep assessment, help setting realistic goals, challenging automatic thinking, learning to identify both positive and negative aspects of events, applying flexibility in interpreting and evaluating, and looking at choices (Scherling, 2006).

Depression is associated with a basic inclination to assign negative meanings to internal thoughts and feelings, relationship difficulties, events and circumstances, and future outcomes (APA, 2004; Scherling, 2006). All of which lead to a sense of hopelessness. The first step in counseling the depressed client is to build hope by collaboratively developing a concept of what is realistically possible in treatment and recovery (Scherling, 2006). Build hope before engaging in any of the above methods (Scherling, 2006).

Bipolar Disorders. Bipolar disorder is also known as manic depression. It is a brain disorder that brings about unordinary mood shifts affecting energy level and ability to function as well (APA, 2004). Everyone has ups and downs, but these shifts are severe. Emmerling, (2008) describes it well. Bipolar disorder may be best seen as a spectrum or continuum. Starting with severe depression on one end, working up through moderate depression, mild depression (the 'blues' when it is temporary and dysthymia when it is chronic) and, balanced mood, then hypomania (mild to moderate mania), then severe mania. Sometimes severe depression or severe mania is accompanied with psychotic symptoms (APA, 2004). Some people experience symptoms of depression and mania together called a mixed episode (APA, 2004).

Signs and symptoms of a mania episode include increased energy; restlessness, excessive euphoric mood; extreme irritability; racing thoughts; rapid speech; distractibility; little sleep needed; unrealistic beliefs of inability and power; poor judgment; spending sprees; increased sex drive; drug abuse; provocative, intrusive, or aggressive behavior; and denial (APA, 2004).

Signs and symptoms of a depressive episode include a lasting sad, anxious, or empty mood, hopelessness; guilt, worthlessness, helplessness; loss of interest or pleasure in life; decreased energy; fatigue; sleeping too much or not enough; chronic pain; and thoughts of death, suicide, or suicide attempts (APA, 2004).

One of the problems with treating bipolar is that a hypomanic stage (mild to moderate) can feel pleasant and even productive, and the individual does not believe anything is wrong (Emmerling, 2008). However, it can cycle to severe mania or depression without treatment (APA, 2004).

The classic form of bipolar disorder involves recurrent manic and depressive episodes and is called bipolar I (APA, 2004). Some people do not experience severe mania, but have milder episodes along with depression; this is called bipolar II (APA, 2004). When four or more cycles occur in one year it is called rapid-cycling which usually occurs later in the illness (APA, 2004).

Best practices with bipolar disorder include a combination of medication and psychosocial treatment (as previously described) over time. Medications called mood stabilizers are usually prescribed. It is important to note that the use of anti-depressants alone with bipolar individuals can trigger mania, therefore they are combined with mood stabilizers when prescribed.

Dysthymic Disorder. Dysthymic Disorder has been touched on in the previous sections. Fundamentally, dysthymia can be more persistent than major depression but less severe (APA, 2004). Common features include fatigue, irritability, poor self esteem, self-pity, social isolation, and clients describe always having been unhappy and depressed (Emmerling, 2008). People do not become as vegetative as they might with major depression. This diagnosis is considered if the client has been depressed every day for most of the day for at least two years (APA, 2004). Dysthymia responds well to anti-depressant medication (Emmerling, 2008).

> *Comment for the Reader:* I am reminded of *Pathways to Recovery* by Ridgway et al. In it, they make a terrific presentation about 'negative self-talk' and the messages that we send ourselves. For most this is an unconscious process. Ways to shift focus to positive impressions are presented. The point is that the shift is based on strengths that the client already possesses, so no one's faking it here, it's all based on existing talents and dreams that may need to be brought up, dusted off, and developed.

Attention-Deficit/Hyperactivity Disorder

ADHD is not a mood disorder, but in its own category as "Attention-Deficit and Disruptive Behavior Disorders." Sometimes, however, ADHD can look like a Manic Disorder and is often misdiagnosed. It is worth including here because a lot of AD and ADHD is seen in dual diagnosis. Let's take a look at common characteristics. According to DSM-IV, inattention can include a lack of attention paid to details, difficulty sustaining attention, appearing not to listen when directly spoken to, lacking follow- through, difficulty organizing tasks or activities, avoiding tasks that require sustained mental effort, often loses things, easily distracted, and is often forgetful. Impulsivity can include: fidgeting, squirming, leaving seat, moving excessively, difficulty engaging in activities quietly, acting driven, and talking excessively. Hyperactivity can include blurting out answers, difficulty waiting turn, and interrupting frequently. Untreated ADHD can be difficult to manage in treatment programs.

Treatment for ADHD

Behavior Therapy that includes rewarding desired behavior with privileges and discouraging other behavior by removing incentives can work with tasks and social skills (Emmerling, 2008). Other treatment includes biofeedback and dietary considerations. Many people do not wish to get involved with medications.

However, research shows that medication provides significant benefits (Emmerling, 2008). Ritalin, Dexidrine Adderall, Vyvanse, and Strattera are used.

In terms of substance use, poor impulse control is a major trigger. People with ADHD have little to no "pause" before making a decision. Cognitive behavioral therapy can help with self-management and social skills. CBT can help the client see the connection between his thoughts and behavior. Negative reinforcement is useful to reduce or eliminate undesired behaviors.

> *Comment for the Reader:* People with ADD/ADHD often have a hard time in treatment programs. First, because we expect them to sit there for 4 hours at a stretch. And, that's a stretch! The other real problem is that their impulsivity in making decisions causes them to relapse before being clean long enough to get stabilized on medications. Then, for some, once they're on medications, they don't like it because it's not as much fun as they were having racing around. There's no easy answer.

Psychoses

If neuroses present distress, dysfunction, and impairment in daily living, psychoses, in addition to the former, present a distortion of an awareness of reality. They have significant impact on people's lives and their families, producing marked dysfunction in one or more areas. Research regarding cause implies limbic system brain dysfunction (Emmerling, 2008).

Schizophrenia. Schizophrenia, according to the DSM-IV, is a relatively long-standing and pervasive disorder. The following is a list of characteristic symptoms: bizarre delusions (unrealistic, unfounded, inaccurate beliefs), hallucinations (auditory, visual, often threatening), disorganized speech and behavior, flat or very inappropriate effect, markedly impaired social and occupational functioning, a confused sense of self, limited insight, dependence conflicts, loose associations, concrete thinking, physical awkwardness, psychomotor disturbances (i.e., catatonic symptoms), and dysphoric moods.

DSM-IV describes three types of schizophrenia. The paranoid type is the most common. It is characterized by systemized delusions and hallucinations and that are related to a theme of grandiosity and persecution, accompanied by anger and suspicion. Schizophreniform disorder may be an indistinguishable form of schizophrenia, but is marked by impaired reality testing, extremely inappropriate behavior, bizarre delusions and hallucinations, incoherence, and catatonia. A Brief Psychotic Disorder is just what it sounds like . . . sudden onset of short-lived symptoms, and a return to previous functioning. Delusional disorder includes five types of delusions: erotomanic type, which involves unrealistic beliefs about a romantic relationship; grandiose type which involves inaccurate beliefs of one's talents or ability; jealous type, which involves an unfounded belief that one's partner is unfaithful; persecutory type, which involves the incorrect belief that others seek to harm oneself – the most common type and; somatic type, which involves unrealistic beliefs about one's body. Schizoaffective Disorder is a more complicated diagnosis. It meets the criteria for a mood disorder (depression or bipolar), but includes delusions and hallucinations. Schizotypal and schizoid personality disorders both include pervasive deficits in interpersonal relationships characterized by cognitive or perceptional distortions

Without a broad analysis of DSM-IV psychotic diagnoses, the above is most pertinent to recognizing psychotic behavior in the various forms that it presents itself.

Treatment for Schizophrenia

Objectives in treatment include reducing or eliminating predominant symptoms as possible, restore clients' awareness of reality, maximizing coping abilities and adjustments to the disorder, helping clients with stressors and traumatic experiences, preventing relapse, and enabling family members (Emmerling, 2008). The counselor must communicate a caring, consistent, and optimistic persona; establish a long-term trusting and therapeutic alliance; collaborate with collateral support; and provide support to the family. Interventions used include supportive counseling; family therapy; education; behavioral therapy (coping skills); and medication, which are almost always indicated for psychotic disorders.

The nature of psychotic disorders with dysfunction and impairment might imply that a harm-reduction approach be taken when addressing substance abuse disorders. Surely, there are times when this is true. It is equally true that there are times when a harm-reduction approach is helpful to the counselor. Quite honestly, this is because some counselors don't believe the client is capable of complete abstinence. This is a mistake. Many clients with psychotic disorders are very capable of maintaining long-term abstinence and recovery, and find their niche in 12-step programs. Many are very capable of understanding that substance usage exacerbates their mental illness.

Comment for the Reader: A word about psychotic disorders and spirituality is appropriate. Because of delusional behavior and hallucinations, spirituality is a tricky thing for these clients. Psychotic clients can have command hallucinations that 'order' them to do things (typically harmful). These commands can be difficult to deviate from without medication, training, and practice. Thus some believe they are receiving messages and/or are talking to spirits and so forth. An important rule of thumb to help clients separate spiritual expression from psychotic symptoms is that anything spiritual in nature is not going to promote harm in any way.

Personality Disorders

I like to think of anxiety and depressive disorders as characteristics that describe a client's distress and dysfunction. Personality disorders are a different animal. They are more pervasive, long-standing, and ingrained. They are the fabric of the personality, whereas anxiety or depression are characteristic of the fabric. While personality disorders certainly affect behavior, it is better described like a temperament and character than attitudes and behavior. As a result, they may be more difficult to treat. According to DSM-I, personality disorders are characterized by maladaptive beliefs and behaviors that include two of the following: the client's perceptions and understanding of themselves and the world; the client's expression and nature of emotions; interpersonal skills; and impulse control. These factors are usually very rigid impacting on the client's distress and dysfunction in significant areas of their lives. Other than schizoid and schizotypal personality types as described in the previous section, personality disorders do not necessarily include psychotic features. Personality disorders vary in terms of impairment and severity, and are very prevalent, but often misdiagnosed. This may be because the counselor may need to know the client for a while before personality patterns emerge.

The DSM-IV groups personality disorders into three clusters. Cluster A – typically guarded or eccentric people, including paranoid, schizoid, and schizotypal personality disorders. Cluster B – typically dramatic, emotional, or unpredictable behavior, including antisocial, borderline, histrionic, and narcissistic personality disorders. Cluster C – anxious and fearful people, including avoidant, dependent, and obsessive-compulsive personality disorders. There is also a personality disorder NOS (not otherwise specified), which encompasses mixed personality disorders and does not fit into any one disorder criteria.

Personality disorders are often seen with other more transient mental disorders and symptoms, such as mood, anxiety, and substance usage (Pervin et al., 2005). Treatment can be more difficult because patterns of behavior are more long-standing and affect social and occupational areas (Pervin et al., 2005). Achieving intimacy is often more difficult for those with personality disorders (Pervin et al., 2005). Pervin et al (2004) continue to describe personality-disorder behavior. There can often be a sense of entitlement and lack of empathy, such that they may violate interpersonal boundaries or act inappropriately. There is a general tendency toward low self-esteem, weak ego strength, and poor impulse control. They may be dependent, self-absorbed, and pessimistic. Underlying fear and rage may be present, and functioning may be impaired on various levels. People with personality disorders may have dysfunctional schemas (belief systems) and maladaptive coping skills, and managing stress and coping with life can present great difficulty. They may have a long history of disappointments and come to see the world as unfriendly.

Treatment for Personality Disorders

Corey (2009) explains that once again, a strong collaborative therapeutic alliance is essential; i.e., empathy, warmth, compassion, acceptance, respect, genuineness, and authenticity. Confrontation or expression of adverse, negative feedback can break the fragile bond that must be developed. Taking sides or arguing with the client may lose them – instead, a supportive approach that allows for trust to gradually increase is effective. Treatment is likely to be long-term and patience is essential. Those with personality disorders are not usually motivated for change, but want the counselor to fix them and/or take care of them. There is often a strong transference that takes place – clients may either become hostile and resistant or dependent and needy, and the counselor must learn to be appropriately available, neither rejecting nor becoming over-involved. Limit setting as necessary, gentle interpretations, rewards, modeling positive behavior, using humor, and appropriate self-disclosure are useful.

Therapy is multifaceted – it can be psychodynamic and cognitive-based, as well as making use of behavioral techniques (Corey, 2009). Progress may be moderate at best because patterns of behavior are ingrained and pervasive in nature, and many with personality disorders leave treatment prematurely. However, if the client remains in treatment and is cooperative, reduced symptoms and improved social functioning and coping skills are likely.

Substance use treatment must be concurrent and on going. It will not be unusual for these clients to have mood and/or anxiety disorders as well, and medication may be necessary before seeing any progress with substance use. These clients are self-medicating, and without some relief either from medications, advancing with coping skills, or successful social interaction, it is not likely persons with personality disorders are going to give up their substances.

Comment for the Reader: Personality disorders are not often diagnosed in treatment programs because they may be more difficult and take time to detect. Often, they present with symptoms that look like various other diagnoses. Over time, the counselor can develop a feel for it; borderline and antisocial personalities are easier to pick up on, for example.

CHAPTER 21

Suicidality/Violence

A training manual for suicidality/violence is beyond the scope and confines of this text. However, the counselor must be aware that dual diagnosis, whether it is substance use with anxiety, depression, or psychotic features, carry with it a higher suicide risk (Seligman, 2005). Risk of suicide is 60-120 times higher for those with co-occurring diagnoses (Nielson et al., 1998). Depending upon the setting you work in, most will come upon it from time to time as many dual clients may have a history of suicidality, either ideation, plan, or attempt, and you could easily find yourself with a suicidal client sitting in your office or group. This chapter will discuss indicators of suicide risk potential and certain counseling skills aimed at a quick – "what to do" – plan.

Regardless of the diagnosis, here are some "Red Flags" to keep in mind. When you have clients with any of these symptoms, it is wise to ask if they think about hurting themselves or other people. These suicidal risk factors include: hopelessness, acute alcohol/drug abuse, inability to feel pleasure (anhedonia), moderate to severe anxiety, insomnia, loss, psychotic, guilt/shame, anniversary of loss, imminent incarceration, panic attacks, chronic pain, serious medical issues, indecisiveness, current intent, current plan, note, previous attempts, # of previous attempts, command hallucinations, diminished concentration, cyclical mood illness, gives away possessions, recent job loss/threat of loss, and imminent loss of parental rights, and of course there may be others. These risk factors are based on statistical research (Scherling, 2008).

Factors for violence risk potential include: history of assault or violence, psychopathy (lack of empathy or care), impulsive, poor anger management, current domestic abuse (victim, abuser, or both), history of abuse (abused child, sexually abused, witnessed abuse), history of arrest/incarceration, access to weapons, history of property destruction, history of cruelty to animals, acute substance abuse, verbal threats, history of fire setting, violent fantasies, imminent incarceration, forced job loss/threat of job loss (Scherling, 2008).

First and foremost, if you are uncertain what to do or feel you are exceeding the boundaries of your skill, bring in a colleague, supervisor, and consultant, or arrange for a referral.

Otherwise, if you have reason to believe the client may be at risk, ask them! Right then and there in your office, in the middle of an intake, and just like that. "Do you think about hurting yourself? Do you want to hurt anybody else?" If the answer is yes, ask, "do you have a plan how you would do that?" This lets you know where they are in their thinking. Suicide/violence may occur when there is no coping available and the client is emotionally overwhelmed. Anxiety and depression are increased and a panic state/disorganization of thought processes may occur (Scherling, 2008). Some counselors are reticent about asking because they fear putting ideas in the client's head. This is a mistake. If a client is not suicidal, it is not likely they will become suicidal by asking them; also it will deter your ability to treat the client.

Scherling (2008), explains that both the client and the counselor may have a resistance to talking about suicidal thoughts. The client may feel they are a weak person and/or be ashamed of themselves. They may feel it is wrong, immoral, and unforgiveable. Some feel the topic cannot be discussed. Clients may be afraid you will think they are crazy and/or lock them up. The client may truly wish to die and does not want anyone to intervene. They may not think you can understand or help.

Scherling (2008) continues discussing the counselor's reservations about discussing suicide. The counselor may feel any of those same things the client is apt to feel. Some counselors may feel suicide is permissible and is an individual issue or that given the circumstances even possesses intrinsic value. They may believe suicide is an innate right, provide dignity, or a way to be reunited with loved ones or God. Sometimes a counselor may just be reluctant to approach the subject with the client because they are uncomfortable with it or how to deal with it.

Herlihy and Corey (1996) discuss the counselor's primary ethical obligations. Nonmaleficence means to do no harm. This means as counselors we have a responsibility to not do anything that might cause harm to the client – even inadvertently. We must not cause harm or potentially cause harm. Furthermore, we must promote beneficence, which means to promote good or wellness, and promote the growth and welfare of our clients. These are the foundation of the code of ethics, so it is imperative that we act responsibly. We cannot ignore a client's vulnerability in these areas of risk for suicidality or violence. We must act.

This means either consulting with an appropriate professional regarding the client, checking out your concerns with the client, and referring the client out if necessary.

There are three components of suicide and risk assessment (Scherling, 2008):

1) Obtaining risk factor information as previously described.
2) Obtaining ideation/plan information at this moment.
3) Applying decision-making and treatment intervention planning.

Schering (2008) describes techniques in interviewing the client for risk assessment include:

1) Obtaining factual information to gain a complete picture of the situation.
2) Be non-judgmental/non-threatening in order to reduce shame; attempt to understand, empathize, and validate clients' feelings (without endorsing risky behavior).
3) Counselor may make gentle assumption that potentially embarrassing or incriminating behavior is occurring at some level.
4) Client may minimize. Counselor can amplify; i.e., how many times have you saved up your medications?
5) Ask specific questions; i.e., if a client indicates a plan to shoot himself, ask if they have also thought about overdosing. Poisoning yourself? Instead of saying, so that's how you would do it? It can come across avoidant, like you really don't want to know because you can't cope with it. Just like when you conduct a substance use history, you wouldn't say . . . so, no other drug use, right? You would say, "have you tried cocaine?" "Have you tried heroin?" Specific questions are harder to lie about than a sweeping question.

Unless you are working in a hospital treatment program, the facility you are working in may not be equipped to deal with the client at this level.

There may be times when it is necessary to call the local Mobile Crisis Team. This is a response unit that combines critical police and emergency hospital personnel. They will make a determination whether or not the client requires hospitalization. Short of that, the client may be able to agree to go to the hospital on his or her own, or with a family member or friend, and agree to have the crisis unit call you when they have arrived. If they fail to do this, you may have to call the police or Mobile Crisis and share your concerns.

In the typical outpatient substance abuse level of care, I am not comfortable with Safety Contracts. They are not a guarantee of safety. If there is a potential for imminent risk, a safety contract is, in my opinion, only a relative and moderate deterrent.

Outpatient management is only warranted if the counselor is able to determine that there is a low risk of suicide; i.e., if the precipitating incident has been removed, the client has a strong support system, and in this case, a safety contract is appropriate (Seligman, 2005).

I will not let someone out of my office until I am convinced that the situation is being handled in the best possible way; this is for the client's well-being as well as for the counselor's liability!

The same goes for a client who is high or intoxicated in your program. If they drove there, they must be prevented from driving home. If they refuse, we have an obligation to inform the authorities of their condition. This is for the client's well-being, the community's welfare, and the agency's/counselor's liability. They may call for a ride or if they are intoxicated, they must turn over their car keys and wait until they are no longer legally drunk. I don't take chances with those who are high on other substances. There is no need to get anxious or raise your voice; the counselor simply informs the client in a business-like fashion that they cannot allow them to drive and why, and let them know your potential course of action. They are welcome to use the phone to call for a ride. I have never had anyone insist on driving and leave regardless. It's as though no matter how angry and upset they get, they know on some level that you are looking out for their best interest. There are times when we are willing to risk our clients being angry with us.

In the case of a potentially violent client, there are several interventions all with the goal of helping the client regain control (*Behavior Management Strategies*, 2003).

1) Provide support and feedback, which can allay the client's fear and hostility.
2) Set limits, firmly and consistently. This lets the client know what the counselor needs from him in order to help him.
3) In a hospital setting, it is sometimes necessary to medicate the client to help him regain control. Seclusion may be necessary, as well.
4) Protect yourself. Verbally encourage the client to talk about his feelings, set limits, show interest, explain the consequences if someone gets hurt. Nonverbally don't turn your back to the client, leave the door open, do not sit between the client and the door, stay seated, keep a distance, leave the room, call for help, pick up a potential weapon, fight back.

Always be sure to document the event well. Typical documentation includes SOAP notes (subjective/objective/assessment/plan) or DAP notes (data, assessment, plan). Integrate all the data and record your reasoning for the action you took. Documentation and communication are major principles in risk management (Scherling, 2008).

Comment for the Reader: My best suggestion is if you are uncertain on any level, of someone's mental status or condition, bring in a colleague or supervisor. You do not want to go home with some nagging concern that you should have done this or that. Listen to yourself. You will know if something is wrong. If you get a fluttering feeling in your stomach, or you feel the need, hone in on your instincts to tune into this person more closely; you get a chill or your "neck hair stands up". . . check it out.

Conclusion

The information in this unit was presented categorically; i.e., diagnosing and treatment for substance abuse and diagnosing and treatment for mental health conditions. When dealing with individuals with co-occurring disorders, these modes are blended together. I believe, at this stage, this is more of an art than science. The counselor must have a repertoire of approaches, methods, and skills that they can utilize with their clients. They must have/develop an intuitive sense regarding what is needed at what time. For example, a chronic substance abuser with an anxiety disorder may need specific how-to skills in terms of coping and relaxation before they are in a place where they can receive and apply recovery information. The depressed client may well need to be stabilized on medications before attempting to deal with family issues in treatment. Some clients may need to do some cleaning up of unfinished business before they will be able to get clean. I know this goes against the order in which recovery is typically approached, but we simply need to do what will work and that may mean working outside the box.

ntended to provide necessary background information ꭗing knowledge of the treatment of co-occurring dis- nuing in the same vein, Unit 6 moves on to talk about drugs and the body.

UNIT 5 Highlights

CH 17: Co-occurring Disorders and Their Treatment

- Approximately 50% of clients have co-occurring disorders
- Integrated treatment poses a unique set of problems due to differences in substance abuse treatment and mental health treatment modalities in the past
- Integrated dual diagnosis treatment utilizes person-centered therapy recovery core values as promoted by SAMSHA/ addresses individual needs, objectives, and attitudes/collaboration between counselor and client in the development of recovery plan/holistic approach/instill hope, confidence, and commitment/goal is client empowerment
- Dual-diagnosed clients have higher rate of relapse and lower quality of life due increased obstacles as both the substance use and other mental health disorder impact and exacerbate each other

CH 18: DSM-IV-TR

- Assists clinical judgment vs. mechanical applications
- DSM is part of comprehensive evaluation/basis for treatment planning
- 3rd party (insurance industry) referential standard for determining level of care

CH 19: Substance Abuse/Substance Dependence

- As a rule of thumb, tolerance and withdrawal separate abuse from dependency

CH 20: Psychiatric Disorders

- Psychiatric disorder = condition causing distress and dysfunction/psychosis = includes delusions and/or hallucinations (auditory/visual/command)
- Anxiety and depression most commonly seen with addiction/alcoholism
- Generalized anxiety disorder (GAD) = excessive worry/physical symptoms
- Post traumatic stress disorder (PTSD) = re-experiencing traumatic event/increased stress/avoidance of triggers and issues
- Panic Disorder = GAD symptoms/re-occurring cycle/focus on stimulus – then physical symptoms – then increased focus on stimulus – then increased physical symptoms
- Agoraphobia = avoidance of places or situations that one cannot escape from easily
- Obsessive compulsive disorder = re-occurring thought, images, impulses/re-occurring distressing behavior/(obsession = thought/compulsion = behavior)
- Social anxiety = high anxiety in situations where one feels evaluated/avoidance
- Treatments include: self-monitoring/relaxing breathing techniques/cognitive restructuring/grounding methods

- Depression = persistent and significant disruption of thought, mood, feeling/inclination to assign negative meanings to events, thoughts, so forth
- Depression treatment includes interpersonal therapy (IPT)/ cognitive behavioral therapy (CBT)/medication
- Bipolar Disorder = severe shifts in mood/manic episodes and depressive episodes
- Bipolar treatment includes psychosocial therapy (IPT/CBT)/ medication
- Dysthymia = more persistent, but less severe than major depression
- Dysthymia treatment/responds well to anti-depressants
- ADHD = AD/difficulty sustaining attention and HD/ blurting out/unable to wait/cannot sit still/interruptions
- ADHD treatment includes behavior modification techniques/medications
- Psychosis/schizophrenia/hallucinations/delusions
- Psychosis treatment/restore awareness to reality/increase coping skills/improve adjustment to illness/deal with stressors/family involvement/medications
- Personality Disorders (PD) = pervasive rather than characteristic disorder/3 clusters/cluster A is guarded – paranoid, schizoid, schizotopal. Cluster B is dramatic, emotional, unpredictable – anti-social, borderline, histrionic, narcissistic. Cluster C is anxious and fearful – avoidant, dependent, obsessive-compulsive /PDs often have anxiety/ depressive components

- Personality Disorder treatment/relies on therapeutic alliance/ psychodynamic approach/CBT/symptomatic medications

CH 21: Suicidality/Violence

- Red Flags for suicidality/hopelessness, acute alcohol/drug abuse, inability to feel pleasure (anhedonia), moderate to severe anxiety, insomnia, loss, psychotic, guilt/shame, anniversary of loss, imminent incarceration, panic attacks, chronic pain, serious medical issues, indecisiveness, current intent, current plan, note, previous attempts, # of previous attempts, command hallucinations, diminished concentration, cyclical mood illness, gives away possessions, recent job loss/threat of loss, and imminent loss of parental rights
- Red Flags for violent behavior/ history of assault or violence, psychopathy (lack of empathy or care), impulsive, poor anger management, current domestic abuse (victim, abuser, or both), history of abuse (abused child, sexually abused, witnessed abuse), history of arrest/incarceration, access to weapons, history of property destruction, history of cruelty to animals, acute substance abuse, verbal threats, history of fire setting, violent fantasies, imminent incarceration, forced job loss/threat of job loss

- Obligation to inquire about suicidal/homicidal ideation
- Suicidal/Homicidal Evaluation
  1) Check for risk factors
  2) Check for ideation/plan to hurt self or others
  3) Consult/Decide on plan for treatment/Interview in non-threatening, non-judgmental manner
- Voluntary vs. involuntary hospitalization/Mobile Crisis Team
- Risk Management/bring others into decision-making process/document all – data, assessment, plan (DAP)

STUDY GUIDE

1) Is your counseling orientation more in line with a traditional mental health approach or a substance abuse approach?
2) What difficulties do you feel may arise in integrated dual-diagnosis counseling?
3) Are there any psychiatric diagnoses, behavior, or populations that you feel might be difficult for you to work with?
4) Are you comfortable working with a suicidal client? If not, what skills do you feel you need to enhance? How can you do that?

References

American Psychiatric Association (2004). *Diagnostic and Statistical Manual* – IV-TR. American Psychiatric Association.

Astals, M.; Domingo-Salvany, A.; Buenaventura, C.; Tato, J.; Vazquez, J.; Martín-Santos, R. et al. (2008). Impact of substance dependence and dual diagnosis on the quality of life of heroin users seeking treatment. *Substance Use & Misuse,* 43(5).

Behavior Management Strategies (2003). State of Connecticut Department of Mental health and Addiction Services/Division of Safety Services.

Bizzarri, J.; Rucci, P.; Vallotta; A., Girelli, M.; Scandolari, A.; Zerbetto, E. et al. (2005). Dual Diagnosis and Quality of Life in Patients in Treatment for Opioid Dependence. *Substance Use & Misuse,* 40(12), 1765-1776. doi:10.1080/10826080500260800.

Blume, A.; Davis, J.; & Schmaling, K. (1999). Neurocognitve dysfunction in dual-diagnosed patients: A potential roadblock to motivating behavior change. *Journal of Psychoactive Drugs* 31(2). 111-115. (see Manning et al.; Levy & Weiss; Horsfall et al.

Corey, G. (1986). *Theory and practice of counseling and psychotherapy* (3rd ed.). Belmont, CA: Wadsworth, Inc.

Corey, G. (2009). *Theory and practice of counseling and psychotherapy* (8th ed.). Belmont, CA: Brooks/Cole.

Delgado, C. (2007). Sense of Coherence, Spirituality, Stress, and Quality of Life in Chronic Illness. *Journal of Nursing Scholarship,* 39(3), 229-34. Retrieved April 18, 2009, from ProQuest *Psychology Journals* database. (Document ID: 1428124701).

Drake, R.E.; McHugo, G.J.; Haiyi, X.; Fox, M.; Packard, P.; Helmstetter, B. (2006). Ten-Year Recovery Outcomes for Clients With Co-occurring Schizophrenia and Substance Use Disorders. *Schizophrenia Bulletin,* 32(3), 464-73. Retrieved April 18, 2009, from ProQuest *Psychology Journals* database. (Document ID: 1072725181).

Emmerling, K. (2008). The DSM-IV-TR. A Handout Presented by Medical Educational Services, Inc./Professional Development Network, Hartford, CT.

Fals-Stewart, W. & Lucente, S. (1994). Treating obsessive compulsive disorder among substance abusers: A guide. *Psycology of Addictive Behaviors.* 8, 14-23.

Finn, P.; Rickert, M.; Miller, M.; Lucas, J.; Bogg, T.; Bobova, L. et al., (2009). Reduced cognitive ability in alcohol dependence: Examining the role of covarying externalizing psychopathology. *Journal of Abnormal Psychology,* 118(1), 100-116.doi:10.1037/a0014656.

Granholm, E.; Anthenelli, R.; Monteiro, R.; Sevcik, J.; & Stoler, M. (2003). Brief Integrated Outpatient Dual-diagnosis Treatment Reduces Psychiatric Hospitalizations. *The American Journal on Addictions,* 12(4), 306-313. Retrieved from PsycINFO database.

Henson, B. (2008). Axis I disorders, dual diagnosis, and health-related quality of life: Results from the national survey on alcohol and related conditions (NESARC) *Dissertation Epidemiologic International,* 68, 5575.

Inaba, D.S.; Cohen, W.E. (2004). *Uppers, downers, all arounders: Physical and mental effects of psychoactive drugs* (5th ed.). Medford, OR: CNS Publications, Inc.

Levy, B. & Weiss, R. (2009). Cognitive functioning in bipolar and co-occurring substance use disorders: A missing piece of the puzzle. *Harvard Review of Psychiatry*, 17(3), 226-230. doi:10.1080/10673220902979870.

Levy, M. & Mann, D. (1987). The special treatment team: An inpatient approach to the mentally ill alcoholic patient. *Journal of Substance Abuse Treatment*, 5, 1–9.

Magura, S.; Cleland, C.; Vogel, H.S.; Knight, E.L.; Laudet. B. (2007). Effects of "Dual Focus" Mutual Aid on Self-Efficacy for Recovery and Quality of Life. *Administration and Policy in Mental Health and Mental Health Services Research*, 34(1), 1-12. Retrieved April 18, 2009, from ProQuest *Psychology Journals* database. (Document ID: 1562965301).

McGovern, M.; Xie, H.; Acquilano, S.; Segal, S.; Siembab, L.; & Drake, R. (2007). Addiction treatment services and co-occurring disorders: The ASAM-PPC-2R taxonomy of program dual diagnosis capability. *Journal of Addictive Diseases*, 26(3), 27-37.doi:10.1300/J069v26n03_04.

Mehr, J. (2001). Introduction to the special issue: Overview of MISA dual diagnosis and treatment. *Psychiatric Rehabilitation Skills*, 5(1), 22-28.

Miller, W. & Rollnick, S. (1991). *Motivational interviewing: Preparing people to change addictive behavior.* NY: Guilford Press.

Minkoff, K. (1987b, October). An innovative clinical model. Paper presented at the Conference on Dual Diagnosis of Psychosis and Addiction: Identification and Treatment, Lexington, MA.

Minkoff, K. (1989). An integrated treatment model for dual diagnosis of psychosis and addiction. *Hospital and Community Psychiatry*, 40, 1031–1036.

Mojtabai, R. (2004). Which Substance Abuse Treatment Facilities Offer Dual Diagnosis Programs? *American Journal of Drug and Alcohol Abuse,* 30(3), 525-536. doi:10.1081/ADA-200032281.

Najavits, L. (2002). *Seeking safety.* NY: Guilford Press.

Nielson, D.A.; Virkumen, M.; Lappalainen, J.; Eggert, M.; Brown, G.; Long, J.; Goldman, D.; & Linoila, M. (1998). A tryptophan hydroxylase gene market for suicidality and alcoholism. *Arhives of General Psychiatry,* 55, 593-602.

Osher, F.C. (2001). Co-occurring addictive and mental disorders. In R.W. Manderscheid & M.J. Henderson (Eds) *Mental health, United States,* 2000. DHHS Publication No. (SMA) ol-3537 Rockville, MD. Center for Mental Health Services.

Pervin, L.; Cervone, D.; & Oliver, J. (2005). Theories of personality. Hoboken, NJ: John Wiley & Sons, Inc.

Pray, M. & Watson, L. (2008). Effectiveness of day treatment for dual-diagnosis patients with severe chronic mental illness. *Journal of Addictions Nursing,* 19(3), 141-149. doi:10.1080/10884600802306008.

Prochaska, J.O.; Diclemente, C.C.; Norcross, J.C. (1992). In search of how people change: applications to addictive behaviors [Electronic Version] *American Psychologist,* 47(9), 1102-1114.

Prochaski, J.; Norcross, J.; & DiClemente, C. (1994). *Changing for good: The revolutionary program that explains the six stages of change and teaches you how to free yourself from bad habits.* NY: William Morrow and Co. Inc.

Prochaski, J.; Gill, P.; Hall, S.; & Hall, M. (2005). Identification and treatment of substance misuse in an inpatient psychiatric unit. *Psychiatric Services.* 56, 347-349.

Rosier, M. (June, 2006). *Co-occurring recovery: Emerging models of integrated care.* Handout Presented at Connecticut Department of Mental Health and Addiction Services Education and Training, Hartford CT.

Scherling, D.H. (2004, October). *Hopeful Conversations: Inspiring Recovery Through Motivational Interviewing.* Handout Presented at Connecticut Department of Mental Health and Addiction Services Education and Training, Middletown, CT.

Scherling, D.H. (2008). *Assessing risk and suicidality; Interviewing skills for clinicians and helpers.* Handout Presented at Connecticut Department of Mental Health and Addiction Services Education and Training, Middletown, CT.

Seligman, L. (2005). *Priniples of psychopathology, diagnosis, and treatment.* Hoboken, N.J.: John Wiley & Sons, Inc.

Singh, J.; Mattoo, S.; Sharan, P.; & Basu, D. (2005). Quality of life and its correlates in patients with dual diagnosis of bipolar affective disorder and substance dependence. *Bipolar Disorders,* 7(2), 187-191. doi:10.1111/j. 1399-5618.2004.00173.x.

Smith Fischer, J. (1999, November).A dual diagnosis treatment program for the courts. (forensic psychology). *Dissertation Abstracts International,* 60, 2368. Retrieved from PsycINFO database.

Tafrate, R. (2004). *Best practices with co-occurring anxiety disorders.* Handout presented at Connecticut Department of Mental Health and Addiction Services Training, Middletown, CT.

Tiet, Q. & Mausbach, B. (2007). Treatments for patients with dual diagnosis: A review. *Alcoholism: Clinical and Experimental Research,* 31(4), 513-536. Retrieved from PsycINFO database.

Timko, C.; Dixon, K.; & Moos, R. (2005). Treatment for Dual-Diagnosis Patients in the Psychiatric and Substance Abuse Systems.*Mental Health Services Research,* 7(4), 229-242. doi:10.1007/s11020-005-7455-9.

Welsh, J.; Buchsbaum, D.; & Kaplan, C. (1993). Quality of life of alcoholics and non-alcoholics: Does excessive drinking make a difference in the urban setting? Quality of Life Research: *An International Journal of Quality of Life Aspects of Treatment, Care & Rehabilitation,* 2(5).

UNIT 6/Drugs and the Body

Introduction

This unit is basic to a working knowledge of how drugs interact with the body and serves to provide an understanding of the physiology of addiction. Hopefully, it is easier to understand why people have such a hard time putting the drug down. This units presents an overview for those of us who do not have a science background. It will discuss drugs, their interaction with the body and the brain, and highlights psychiatric medications.

CHAPTER 22

Major Drugs and How They Affect the Body

A psychoactive drug is any substance that directly alters the normal functioning of the central nervous system (Inaba & Cohen, 2000). For our purposes, there are four categories for psychoactive drugs: stimulants, depressants, psychedelics, and others (inhalants, sports drugs, psychiatric medications). Sources for this section are Inaba and Cohen (2000), Meyer and Quenzer (2005), and Mulready (2008).

Stimulants include cocaine (freebase, crack), amphetamines (speed, meth, crank, ice, Ritalin, diet pills) and others, such as caffeine and nicotine. The central nervous system is stimulated increasing energy, heart rate, and blood pressure, as well as insomnia and decreased appetite. Frequent and/or excessive use will deplete the body of energy. The user may be at risk for heart, blood vessel, and seizure problems. Stimulant use can make someone feel more confident, excited, and outgoing and talkative. There can be a rush or ecstatic feeling. The user may also feel jittery, anxious, and aggressive. Continued use can cause paranoia, an inability to experience pleasure, mental confusion, and may even look like psychosis.

Depressants may be put into four categories. Opiates include heroin, morphine, codeine, oxycodone (oxycontin, percacet), hydrocodone (vicodin), methadone, hydromorphine (dilaudid), and meperidine (Demerol). Sedative-hypnotics include benzodiazepines (alprazolam – xanax, diazepam – valium, clonazepam - klonipin); barbituates (butalbital, zolpidem – ambient). Alcohol, of course, includes beer, wine, and hard liquor. Some people are surprised to find alcohol in this category and think it is a stimulant because of how it makes them feel. There are others: antihistamines (benedryl), muscle relaxants, and look-alike sedatives. Depressants slow down the heart rate and respiration, relax muscles, affect coordination, dull the senses, produce sleep, slur speech, cause sexual dysfunction and reduce pain. They can also cause constipation, nausea, pinpoint (constricted) pupils, respiratory depression, and coma. Initially, depressants induce euphoria, relax the individual and lower inhibitions.

Psychedelics or hallucinogens include LSD, psilocybin mushrooms, peyote (mescaline), MDMA (ecstasy), marijuana, hashish, ketamine, and PCP. These are all substances that can cause perceptual distortions, illusions, delusions, and hallucinations. Initially, mushrooms and peyote can cause nausea and dizziness. Cannabinoids increase appetite and cause bloodshot eyes. LSD can raise blood pressure and produce sweating. People take psychedelics because they distort and intensify sensory perception.

Inhalants can be a gas or liquid which is inhaled and includes solvents; i.e., glue, gasoline, paints, household sprays, nitrates; i.e, amyl and butyl, and anesthetics; i.e., nitrous oxide. These are depressants and can cause dizziness, slurred speech, uncoordination, drowsiness, stupor, coma, and asphyxiation. They also cause excitement, mental confusion and irritability.

Sports drugs are performance-enhancing drugs; i.e., anabolic-androgenic steroids. Some include stimulants, human growth hormones; herbal supplements, painkillers, beta-blockers, and diuretics. Basically, steroids increase muscle mass and strength and can provide increased confidence. However, they can cause high blood pressure, acne, shrunken testes or masculinization in women, and aggression.

Psychiatric medications are used to rebalance irregular brain chemistry that has contributed to mental health disorders. They include antipsychotics, such as risperidol, zyprexa, thorazine, and many others. Antipsychotics manipulate dopamine to control schizophrenia. Antidepressants such as prozac, Zoloft, paxil, lexepro, wellbutrin, and many others manipulate brain chemicals like seratonin, and work to elevate mood. Antianxiety medications like xanax, seraquel, buspar, inderal, and others manipulate brain chemicals like GABA and reduce anxiety-producing thoughts. There can be a wide variety of side effects, including heart, blood, and skeletal- muscle systems. However, the mental and emotional effects are more significant.

Comment for the Reader: We, as counselors, become primarily concerned with relapse prevention, triggers to use, and coping strategies to avoid use, and may not have the scientific background to understand the different types of drugs and their effects on the body. A cursory study and basic understanding is sufficient in most cases. In other instances when a more detailed explanation is needed, it provides the opportunity for further knowledge and experience.

CHAPTER 23

THE BRAIN

Sources for this section are Inaba and Cohen (2000), Meyer and Quenzer (2005), and Mulready (2008). In this chapter, we will learn that the brain and nervous system control every function of our body, thus when a substance arrives at the brain, it alters the way we function. Furthermore, our brain stores information about those drugs, which is how addictions can be formed. Psychoactive drugs are administered to the body by inhalation, injection, mucous membrane absorption, oral ingestion, or contact absorption. They are absorbed through body tissue, which emits it into the bloodstream through the circulatory system. The drug then crosses into the central nervous system (which includes the brain) where it will do one of several things: it may cause an effect, it may be ignored, it may be absorbed, or it may be transformed. Further elaboration on these processes goes beyond the scope of this book. What's important to note however, is how drugs are administered and how by making their way to the brain, can alter the way we function.

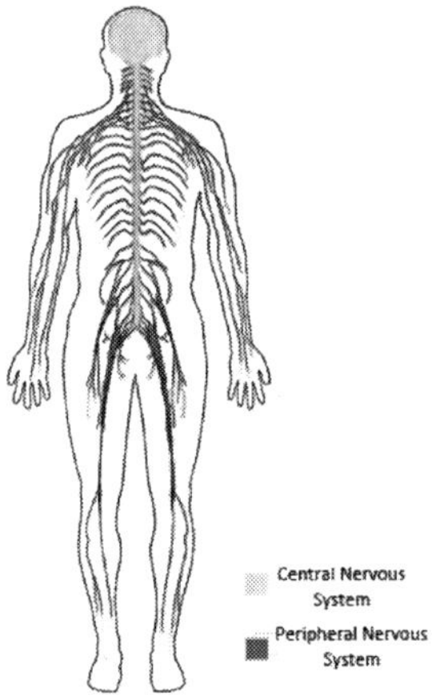

Figure 22.1 – Depicted above is the human nervous system. The central nervous system consists of the brain and spinal cord. The peripheral nervous system consists of the nerves connecting to and from the central nervous system, and the rest of the body (i.e., muscles, organs).

In order to understand how our brain and nervous system function, we must learn how the brain and nervous system communicate with our body. We will start by discussing the nervous system. First, there are two parts to the nervous system, the peripheral nervous system (autonomic and somatic systems) and the central nervous system (brain and spinal cord), see *figure 22.1*. The peripheral nervous system is called such because it connects the "peripherals" of our body (our limbs/extremities and organs) to our central nervous system, which is our control center. The autonomic aspect of the peripheral nervous system controls involuntary body functions, or, everything in our body that we don't have to think about; i.e., digestion, heart rate, or our reflexes. In other words, it keeps our body running subconsciously. The somatic aspect of the peripheral nervous system is more in charge of voluntary control, such as contracting muscles to stand up or walk. It is important to note, however, that voluntary doesn't mean the movement can't be reflexive, or seem to have very little "conscious" thought involved. The central nervous system, the brain and spinal cord, receive information from the peripheral nervous system, analyzes it, and sends action messages accordingly to muscles and organs. To best describe this process, you could imagine a mosquito landing on your arm. You feel the mosquito land, which sends a signal through the peripheral nervous system to your central nervous system, where you decide you don't want the mosquito there. The central nervous system then tells your free hand to slap the mosquito, or less maliciously, shoo it away.

As mentioned before, the central nervous system consists of the brain and spinal cord. If our nervous system is like a system of roads carrying information back and forth, then the spinal cord is the main interstate, where the vast majority of nerves converge and then attach to the brain. The brain then, of course, is our town hall, our government. The brain is what truly dictates our actions, consciously and unconsciously. Our brain also consists of two key parts, the old brain and the new brain. Let's take a look (see *figure 22.2 on next page*).

The old brain or primal brain consists of the brain stem, cerebellum, and mesocortex – which contains the limbic system and is the emotion center. The old brain regulates physiological functions, experiences emotions and cravings, and holds survival memories. The essential thing to understand about the old brain is that it is the center for our instincts. Although they may often trigger "voluntary" muscular responses, signals from the old brain shoot right past our conscious thoughts or reasoning, and turn right into action. That's not to say that the old brain can't learn new tricks, it just takes time. The old brain stores all of our routines – once something is practiced enough we hardly need any conscious thought to conduct the old routine. For example, have you ever driven to work and, upon arrival, realize that you don't remember any details from your trip? This is because the route to work is hardwired in your old brain; you don't need to think much to get there. Of course, if something new happens, like there is unexpected traffic, the new brain might kick in to consciously assess a better route or detour. You also would more likely remember the corresponding details of that trip to work.

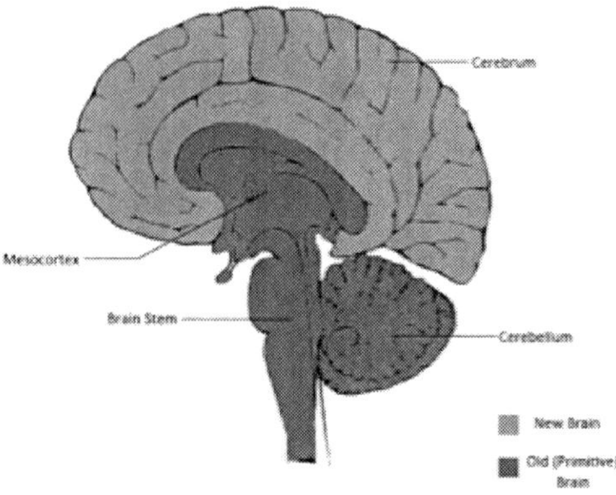

Figure 22.2 – Depicted above is a bisection of the human brain. The new brain is in charge of conscious thought and cognitive reasoning, the old brain is in charge of our more primitive and routinized functions. Within the mesocortex is the limbic system, which is the human emotion center.

Just like your old brain remembers daily routines, the old brain retains addiction memories – the experience and how it felt. These memories can be triggered over and over again and create the desire to use the drug. With the complex network of signals that operate in our brain, there is a very broad spectrum of associations, or "triggers," that could elicit such a response. In other words, there are a lot of things that the old brain remembers about the experience that we may or may not consciously think about, but many various emotions or physical feelings could remind the brain of the drug's effects, and thus one starts desiring it.

The new brain or neocortex, consists of the cerebrum. It processes information from the old brain, various areas of the new brain, or from the peripheral nervous system. More importantly for us, however, is understanding that the new brain is where our cognition comes from. It is where we contemplate, assess, reason, and make decisions; it is the center for our conscious thoughts. Where the old brain acts on impulse, the new brain acts more slowly, allowing time for consideration and reasoning before generating action. To put it into perspective, conscious reaction takes about 1.5 to 2 seconds, whereas an instinctive reaction from the old brain is about 10 times faster. Going back to the Freudian analogy, one could say that the new brain produces the voices of our ego and super ego, which apply more reason to what they tell us in an attempt to organize our thoughts and regulate our behavior. Where some deviation and complications arise, is in establishing whose voice is louder, the old brain or the new brain? Now that we know the old brain is where we store our addiction memories, and that our new brain controls our conscious thought, clearly the volume of their voices play a hand in our decision to use or not. Or maybe even whether we're addicted or not.

Comment for the Reader: The old brain generally dictates over the new brain. In other words, when there is a craving to use a drug (from the old brain), it will win out over the voice of reason (from the new brain). Part of this can be attributed to speed and impulsivity; as we mentioned, the old brain acts more quickly. Also, because the old brain acts at a subconscious level, the new brain may not even get the chance to reconsider an action before taking it! This represents the essence of the paramount conflict the addict/alcoholic goes through when trying to control their usage.

The old brain holds the reward and reinforcement center. This area produces a surge of satisfaction when a bodily or environmental need is met. Drug usage affects this center directly. The new brain knows that there are societal restraints prohibiting drug use, that it is costly, is not in their best interest, is unhealthy, creates multiple problems, creates multiple consequences, and so on and so on. The longer someone uses, the stronger the "do it again" message is from the old brain. Also, there are switches that allow for changes in the way genes work. Psychoactive drugs turn some switches on and some off and this can change our behavior.

Psychoactive drugs can also affect the nerve cells of the brain and spinal cord (the central nervous system) and alter the way messages are transmitted to appropriate systems of the body (muscles, organs, nervous, skeletal, circulatory, respiratory, digestive, excretive). In order to understand these alterations, we must develop a basic understanding of how the nervous system communicates with the rest of the body. Neurochemicals, called neurotransmitters, act as messengers between nerve cells. There are several major transmitters. The most common ones that most people are familiar with are serotonin, norepinephrine, and dopamine. Serotonin helps control mood stability, including depression, anxiety, appetite, sleep, and sexual activity. Norepinephrine (and epinephrine) function as stimulants when activated by a demand for energy. They also affect motivation, hunger, attention span, confidence, and alertness. Dopamine helps to regulate fine motor muscular activity, emotional stability, satiation, and the reward/reinforcement center.

Nerve cells, or neurons, communicate with each other at the synapse, which is where two nerve cells meet (see *figure 22.3 on next page*). Neurons have vesicles containing neurotransmitters like the ones described above. When the neuron receives a signal it releases the neurotransmitter to be picked up by the other nerve cell's receptors. A receptor is the spot on a cell where the chemical message in a neurotransmitter carries out its main effect. It is like a key slipping into a lock. Once enough of the receptors have been activated, the signal will pass to the next neuron in the same fashion. Once the signal is passed on the neurotransmitters leave the synapse in one of two ways. One is, they can be destroyed by an enzyme designed to do so. Two, in many cases the neurotransmitters are recycled by being reabsorbed by the original neuron. This process is called 'reuptake' and will be important when we discuss psychotropic medication in the next section. Also, each neuron transferring information is constantly adapting its sensitivity by either increasing or decreasing the number of neurotransmitter receptor cites. If a neuron is subjected to low levels of a given transmitter, that nerve cell will respond by increasing/decreasing (up-regulating/down-regulating) the number of receptors available. Drugs can modify or mimic the way these neurotransmitters function and thus cause physical, mental, and emotional effects.

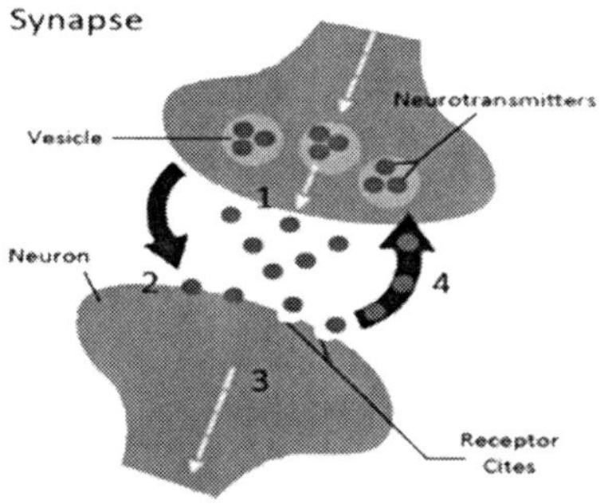

Figure 22.3 – Depicted above is a synapse between two neurons, and the four primary steps involved in neurotransmission. 1) A signal travels down the neuron and releases neurotransmitters, 2) Neurotransmitters are received by the receptor sites on the next neuron, 3) The signal is passed on by the recipient neuron, 4) Most of the neurotransmitters are reabsorbed by the original neuron. Note: Enzymes that destroy additional neurotransmitters are not depicted.

Psychoactive drugs work because they mimic or disrupt naturally occurring chemicals in the body that have specific receptors. Thus, a psychoactive drug cannot create effects if there is not a natural counterpart in the body (because they work like keys in locks as explained before). Often, people seem to be drawn to certain drugs that correlate to their particular neurotransmitters in balance.

In addition to these effects, phenomena like tolerance, physical dependence, psychological dependence, and withdrawal, will determine the nature of an individual's addictive reaction to the psychoactive drugs.

CHAPTER 24

DETOXIFICATION, WITHDRAWAL, AND POST-ACUTE WITHDRAWAL SYNDROME

Sources for this section are Inaba and Cohen (2000); Meyer and Quenzer (2005); Mulready (2008) and Doweiko, (2009). When drug/alcohol use has stopped, there is a period of readjustment so that the body can heal from the effects of the drug/alcohol usage. Many people don't feel quite right for some time, perhaps even months. They complain of anxiety, depression, sleep difficulty, irritability, and agitation. The type and extent of symptoms is related to the type of drug(s) used, the amount and frequency, and may require hospitalization and detoxification.

Opiate users may experience a 7-10 day period of withdrawal; other prescription drug users; i.e., benzodiazepines may be longer. Withdrawal is physically uncomfortable and may require medication. It is highly recommended that physically dependent users are medically monitored. The user may also experience insomnia, depression, anxiety and trouble cognitively, and with concentration. Successful withdrawal is a significant hurdle overcome. Basically, physical recovery is gradual and is similar to alcohol.

Stimulant users experience significant cravings, depression, difficulty sleeping, increased appetite, low energy, and trouble with concentration. Physical withdrawal is not as severe as opiate or alcohol users. However, craving and depression can be significant. Stimulant users often start to feel better in the next few weeks.

Many do not believe that marijuana produces withdrawal symptoms and are surprised to see it included in this type of discussion. The quality/potency of cannabis has significantly increased over the years and users experience withdrawal symptoms, including restlessness, depression, sleeplessness, appetite loss, irritability and agitation, and possible increased aggression. Cannabis dependence may be accompanied with strong cravings, especially when there is an intense psychological dependence. Cannabis is fat-soluble, causing it to remain in the body for months, and its effects may be felt for some time. Speech, memory, decision-making abilities and other cognitive functions will continue to be affected during this period.

Alcohol used in large amounts produces the most severe withdrawal, including tremors, shakes, depression, emotionality, nausea, irritability, and memory and concentration difficulty. Often people require detox which can last 3-5 days with continued complaints for several weeks. The next 4 weeks or so the body and brain are still recovering, and even though physical withdrawal is complete, it takes time to get used to be without alcohol. Cognitive functioning continues to be affected; i.e, thinking, memory, and concentration, along with nervousness and anxiety.

For some people, getting back to 'normal' takes more time – perhaps 1-4 months. This is called post-acute-withdrawal syndrome (PAWS) or protracted withdrawal. They may experience a number of nagging symptoms cognitively and with mood. Emotionality, difficulty thinking, low energy, and a lack of enthusiasm continues as the brain heals. Effects may be subtle, but felt nonetheless, and are a result of brain chemistry. If relapse is averted, these symptoms will pass. A one day at a time approach is most useful. Getting past post-acute withdrawal syndrome is a tremendous hurdle. Generally, after about 3 months, the brain has mostly healed allowing the addict/alcoholic to get on with the business of recovery.

CHAPTER 25

MEDICATIONS

Sources for this section are Inaba and Cohen (2000), Meyer and Quenzer (2005), and Mulready (2008) and Doweiko (2009).

Antipsychotic medications are prescribed for the management of psychotic symptoms (i.e., voices, hallucinations, thought disorders, delusions, and accompanying anxiety and depression). There are off-label (other things they work for) uses as well (mood management, anxiety. Anti-psychotic medications are categorized as conventional or typical vs. atypical drugs. Basically, the atypical medications represent a new generation of drugs that are safer and offer more advantages and less side effects than their counterparts. There is much controversy and research on the subject. High potency conventional antipsychotics (high potency means less drug is needed; low potency means higher dosages needed) include Haldol, Prolixin, Navane, and Stelazine. Moderate potency antipsychotics include Trilaphon, Moban, and Loxitane. Low-potency antipsychotics include Thorazine, Mellaril, and Serentil. Typical antipsychotics bind to dopamine receptors. This means that they prevent dopamine from being transmitted to the receptors, which decreases the effect of dopamine on the brain. This seems to reduce the symptoms of psychoses (delusions, hallucinations, and thought disorder).

Atypical antipsychotics include Clozaril, Risperdal, Zyprexa, Seraquel, Geodon, and Abilify. These block dopamine and serotonin receptors. They are known to reduce psychotic symptoms, as well as to increase social functioning, motivation, and ability to experience pleasure, which contribute toward a positive quality of life.

Antidepressants. Antidepressants are used for the treatment of depression and often for anxiety. There are three categories of antidepressants: Selective Serotonin Reuptake Inhibitors (SSRI), Tricyclic antidepressants, and Monamine Oxidase Inhibitors (MAOI).

SSRIs, (Prozac, Zoloft, Celexa, Paxil, Luvox, and Lexapro) on the whole have less side effects than tricyclics and MAOIs. They are also very helpful treating obsessive-compulsive disorder, panic disorder, and eating disorders. SSRIs increase the amount of serotonin available to the nervous system (blocking the reuptake increases transmission). The most common side effects include insomnia, nausea, diarrhea, headache, and nervousness, and are considered to be mild. However, it usually takes 2-4 weeks for the full effect to be felt. Many of the side effects subside. If SSRIs are used with illicit drugs that also stimulate serotonin, "serotonin syndrome" can occur due to excessive serotonin, which causes elevated temperature, shivering, tremors, mental changes, and nervous system instability.

Tricyclic antidepressants used to be the preferred treatment for depression until the newer SSRIs came out. Tricyclics include imipramine and desipramine. They block the reabsorption of serotonin and norepinephrine and increase the transmission of both neurotransmitters. These drugs are also dangerous for the heart if mixed with illicit drug use.

MAOIs, which include Nardil, Parnate, Marplan, are strong drugs that block the enzyme (Monamine Oxidase) that metabolizes norepinephrine and serotonin, and which raises the levels of these neurotransmitters. MAOIs have potentially dangerous side effects (high blood pressure, headaches, and others) and need to be monitored carefully. Combined use with illicit stimulants and depressants can be fatal.

All of the antidepressant categories basically do the same thing, that is, increase serotonin or serotonin and norepinephrine, but they do it in different ways.

Medications for Bipolar Disorder. Bipolar medications are used to regulate mood. These medications include three categories: anti-mania drugs, such as Lithium, Seraquel, Zyprexa, and Risperdal; anti-depressants (previously described); and anti-convulsants such as Tegretol, Neurontin, Lamictal, Topomax, and Depakote.

Lithium is a salt that is also found naturally in the body; its function is unknown. It acts as a mood stabilzer. Levels of lithium must be monitored because too little lithium can produce a relapse in symptoms and too much can be toxic, producing tremors, thirst, increased urination, diarrhea, vomiting, drowsiness, weakness and coordination problems, and seizures. The therapeutic level is very close to the toxic level.

Antipsychotics like Zyprexa, Risperdol, and Seraquel are used for bipolar disorder because they help with sleep, anxiety, and/or agitation. They also work with delusions and hallucinations, which occur with manic behavior. They block dopamine and raise serotonin to increase mood and cognitive functioning, as well as decreasing depression and mania. They are all associated with significant weight gain with the exception of Geodon. Abilify increases seratonin and dopamine as well as decreasing serotonin at other receptor sites.

Anti-convulsant medications can prevent seizure by suppressing the neurons that start seizures. It is for this reason that it is useful for treating dysfunctional anxiety. Also, anti-convulsants stabilize mood and rapid-cycling.

It is important to note that the use of anti-depressants alone with bipolar individuals can trigger mania, therefore they are combined with mood stabilizers when prescribed.

Anxiety Medication. Anxiety medications are used to manage the distress from anxiety. Benzodiazepines (Xanax, Valium, Klonopin) are widely used, but must only be used with substance users if nothing else works, as they are highly addictive. Benzodiazepines were considered a safe substitute for barbituates and less dangerous in overdose, but certainly not the first choice for the addict. Buspar is used a lot and is a serotonin modulator. Today, many of the SSRI antidepressants (Paxil, Lexapro) are used for anxiety. Anti-psychotics like Seraquel and Risperidol are used as well.

ADHD Medications. It seems that many stimulants in small doses assist to focus attention and control hyperactivity. It is theorized that dopamine depletion is a cause of ADHD, and amphetamines and similar drugs force the release of dopamine and prevent its reuptake. Ritalin, Dexedrine, Adderall, and Vyvanse are used for ADHD.

Addiction Medications

Alcohol. Benzodiazepines are the medication of choice for alcohol withdrawal – chlordiazepoxide (Librium) or diazepam (Valium). Disulfirum (Antabuse) is used for treating alcohol dependence. It deters drinking because the individual will get ill if they do drink. Ondansetron (Zofran) reduces the desire to drink as well as the pleasant effects of alcohol if one does drink. Naltrexone hydrochloride is shown to reduce alcohol cravings in some instances. However, it can reduce the effects of alcohol if used. Acamprosate (Campral) has received widespread acceptance to reduce the desire to drink. Topirmate (Topamax) blocks the effects of alcohol also, and thus reduces the desire to drink.

Opiates. Naltrexone hydrochloride, also sold as Vivetrol, is an opiate blocker and is used to treat opiate dependence. Methadone, also, is a big gun and produces significant dependence. Buprenorphine (suboxone) has become very popular because it is safer than methadone. Suboxone can aid the individual to withdraw safely from opiates and then block its effects. It can precipitate withdrawal effects if abused in high doses because it will then limit its own analgesic potential.

Stimulants. Currently, there is not a medication for stimulant dependence. However, antabuse can produce dysphoric effects if used with cocaine and can therefore be a deterent.

Cannabis. Currently, there is not a medication for cannabis dependence.

CONCLUSION

This unit provided a basic understanding of how drugs interact with the body. Central to this discussion is an understanding of thc brain and neurotransmitters. Also, it may be useful to think of a psychiatric medication as another tool in the toolbox.

In Unit 7, we go into a discourse of different ways to be in recovery from co-occurring disorders. So far, we have just alluded to means other than AA. The next unit will spell it out. Included in this unit is stages of spirituality research which has been demonstrated to enhance recovery and many feel is essential to recovery.

UNIT 6 Highlights

CH 22: Major drugs

- 4 major classifications = stimulants/depressants/psychedelics/other – inhalants, sports drugs, psychiatric medications

CH 23: The Brain

- Peripheral Nervous System/controls involuntary body functions, relays sensory information and sends messages to muscles and organs, receives messages from the central nervous system.
- Central Nervous System/the brain and spinal cord/receives information from the peripheral nervous system, analyzes it, and sends action messages accordingly to muscles and organs.
- Old Brain/limbic system/emotion center/dictates over new brain/reward and reinforcement center.
- New brain/speak, reason, remember.
- Drugs affect CNS/alter messages to body systems.
- Drugs mimic or disrupt naturally occurring chemicals in the body.
- Neurotransmitters = serotonin/norepernephrine/dopamine/sends chemical messages to receptors/determines mood, sleep, appetite, sexual activity, reward center.

CH 24: Detoxification, Withdrawal, and Post-Acute Withdrawal Syndrome

- Detoxification usually takes 3-5 days.
- Readjustment/healing symptoms may last up to 4 months (Post Acute Withdrawal Syndrome).

CH 25: Psychiatric Medications

- Psychotropic/typical – conventional vs. atypical considered safer/high potency vs. low potency/modulates dopamine/ reduces psychiatric symptoms.
- Anti-depressants/three categories of anti-depressants/ Selective Serotonin Reuptake Inhibitors (SSRI)/Ticyclic antidepressants/Monamine Oxidase Inhibitors (MAOI)/ all modulate serotonin and noreprenephrine, but in different ways/regulates mood.
- Bipolar medications/anti-mania drugs/anti-convulsant drugs/ stabilize mood/reduce cycling
- Anxiety Medications/benzodiazapines less dangerous than barbituates – both highly addictive/SSRIs and anti-psychotics also used/better for addict/alcoholic.
- ADHD Medications/stimulants assist to focus attention and control hyperactivity
- Addiction medications/alcohol – naltrexone, antabuse, topomax, and campral/for opiates – naltrexone, methadone, and suboxone/for cocaine – naltexone

Study Guide

1) Describe how drugs impact on the brain.

References

Doweiko, H. (2009). Concepts of chemical dependency (7th ed.). U.S.: Brooks/Cole.Inaba, D.S.; Cohen, W.E. (2004). *Uppers, downers, all arounders: Physical and mental effects of psychoactive drugs* (5th ed.). Medford, OR: CNS Publications, Inc.

Mulready, P. (2008). *Drugs and the brain.* A Handout presented at Connecticut Department of Mental Health and Addiction Services, Plainville, CT.

Meyer, J. & Quenzer, L. (2005). *Pychopharmocology.* Sutherland, MA: Sinauer Associates.

UNIT 7/Recovery Theory

Introduction

We have made it clear that AA and 12-Step programs are not the only way to be in recovery. In this unit, we discuss five means by which people may achieve recovery. It is important to note that those in recovery refer to themselves as 'recovering' as opposed to 'recovered.' This is indicative of the fact that recovery is an on-going process and we are never done with it. It also reminds us that the addict must always have a vigilance against relapse as one is never 'cured' or 'safe' from re-occurrence of addiction and its consequences. Unit 7 includes research regarding Stages of Spirituality which many, in and outside of AA, believe to be quite instrumental in the recovery process.

CHAPTER 26

Five Ways to Recover

Contrary to popular belief, in the 60s, 70s, 80s, and 90s, AA and 12-Step offshoot programs were not the only way to recover. Everyone with a substance use problem got pigeonholed into being addict or alcoholic. If you landed in a treatment facility, not only were you automatically an addict or alcoholic, but AA was the only answer. If you didn't agree that you were drug/alcohol dependent, you were in denial. And, if you didn't like AA or think it was for you, you hadn't reached your bottom yet. Because if you did, you'd be willing to go to any lengths for your recovery.

AA is certainly the most widely accepted and utilized means of recovery, but we are no longer naïve enough to think that it is the only way. First of all, not everyone fits the medical model. There are various stages of drug use and clearly not everyone in treatment programs is chemically dependent. Furthermore, there is more than one way to deal with a drug problem.

For some people, substance use may be symptomatic of another problem. There may be a situational crisis, an unresolved issue, or drug use may be in response to anxiety and/or depression. But, all those can lead to chemical dependency, you say. Yes, that is true, but we can try to intervene before it gets to those proportions. We have moved past a 'one size fits all' mode of treatment, thank goodness. We know more now.

We tend to believe, now, that the client has the capacity and ability to solve their own problems. We providers have moved from the role of expert, director, authoritarian, to working collaboratively with the client and respecting their perspective. We have learned to meet them where they are, instead of harshly confronting them to be where we thought they were. As a result, we have adopted new ways of thinking about Recovery, new methods to working with the clients, and new strategies to prevent relapse. In this section, we will explore these new ideas.

12-STEP PROGRAMS

12-Step Programs. Alcoholics Anonymous and all the offshoots – Narcotics Anonymous, Cocaine Anonymous, Al-Anon, Al-Ateen, Nar-Anon, and so forth remain very powerful, successful, and prevalent programs. I suspect, in addition to providing a means to recovery, that they are so effective due to a magic ingredient. The magic ingredient is Fellowship. In the NA preamble, it states, ". . . the therapeutic value of one addict helping another is without parallel." Long-standing members find that while AA may not have an answer for every problem that arises, it will get them through any problem that may arise. Over a million members (AA alone) look forward to sharing their sorrows and joys with each other. Pain is shared and happiness is multiplied.

Working the Steps. The twelve promises in Alcoholics Anonymous tell us that "if we are painstaking about this phase (working the Steps) of our development, we will be amazed before we are halfway through. We are going to know a new freedom and a new happiness. We will not regret the past nor wish to shut the door on it. We will comprehend the word 'serenity' and we will know peace. No matter how far down the scale we have gone, we will see that our experiences can benefit others. That feeling of uselessness and self-pity will disappear. We will lose interest in selfish things and gain interest in our fellows. Self-seeking will slip away. Our whole attitude and outlook on life will change. Fear of people and economic insecurity will leave us. We will intuitively know how to handle situations, which used to baffle us. We will suddenly realize that God is doing for us what we could not do for ourselves. Are these extravagant promises? We think not. They are being fulfilled among us – sometimes quickly, sometimes slowly. They will always materialize if we work for them."

It's a pretty powerful message that many, many people provide testimony to. It is a result of working the 12 Steps. Let's take a closer look at them. There are many published Step Guides. The Steps should typically be worked by attending Step Meetings with the help of a sponsor or another who is seasoned in recovery and well versed with the Steps. The counselor can supplement and support this in the office if the client is looking for more structure and/or clinical approach. I have done Steps 1-4 in the office with clients with the use of Step guides, have used similar clinical framework as Yalom offers in Chapter 10, and tied in my knowledge of the client. The counselor can provide a more in-depth perspective for the client. The following will highlight some key areas.

It must be remembered that working the Steps is a spiritual process. Some people are turned of by anything relating to the idea of God, spirituality, and religion. Generally, this is due to misconception. First, AA says to "take what you want and leave the rest." Second, AA is a spiritual program, not religious (see spirituality/religion chapter for differences). Third, the concept of God is one of our understanding (Step 3 on Page 126 provides a list of 'synonyms' for 'God'), not anybody else's. These things may need to be discussed with the client. Most everyone pursues spiritual concepts in one manner or another, but knows it by a different name. Anyone who seeks to grow; improve; find joy; appreciate their family, nature, and life; reach their goals; be all they can be; be the best person they are capable of; help people; be kind; and so forth – has spirituality.

Step 1. We admitted that we were powerless over our addiction and life became unmanageable. This Step must be understood if one is going to be in recovery. Addicts and alcoholics have an "X" factor (Springborn, 1992). This means that they respond differently to alcohol and other drugs than 'earth people' (people who are not addicted)do. It has not yet been scientifically determined what exactly is different or why. Basically, there are currently too many factors with too many variables, to make such a determination as to why some people get addicted and others don't. For this reason, it is called an 'X' factor (Springborn, 1992). Nonetheless, the implication is that this is not a fault that people need to feel guilty about. One cannot control the constitution of the body, but we know that this X factor affects addicts/alcoholics physically and psychologically. Having said this, there is an inherent need to be responsible for one's recovery. Staying clean and sober has to come first and the individual must let go of any reservations (Alcoholics Anoymous, 2002; Narcotics Anonymous, 1984).

As indicated in Chapter 11, many people initially get hung up on the word 'powerless.' We just don't want to admit that something has control over us. Regardless of the consequences we have endured, we still like to hold out that we can control our use of drugs. For many, it is much easier to see that our life has become 'unmanageable.' One look at our finances, relationships, legal issues, occupational pitfalls, medical problems, and our demeanor and appearance, tells us that life has gotten away from us, to put it delicately. Often then, people are more willing to recognize that they cannot control the use of drugs/alcohol. Whew! Where does that leave us?

Step 2. We came to believe that a power greater than ourselves could restore us to sanity. Most are left in a void at this point. Where do I go from here? What do I do now? A good start on Step 1 will most always leave one exhausted at their own resources, and depleted. This is a good thing. How is that possible? For all appearances, on an unguided tour, the individual has just been stripped of any self-esteem and self-respect that may have been left. This is merely a smokescreen. It is a cloud of smoke that conceals the spiritual awareness that has just begun to emerge at that very same moment. Spiritual awareness begins to displace the junkyard left behind. What a relief! Sanity means sound mental health. Sound mental health means healthy, robust, competent, sensible, upright, and honorable, sustaining and enduring. And that's where we are going. Step 2 is "the difference between getting sober and living sober" (Springborn, 1992, p. 3). Critics may suggest that Step 2 indicates that the addict/alcoholic cannot rely on themselves. On the contrary, now is the time to look inward. Step 2 is "an inside job" (Springborn, 1992, p. 12). The Step is considered necessary for any ongoing recovery (Alcoholics Anonymous, 2002; Narcotics Anonymous, 1984).

Step 3. We made a decision to turn our life and will over to the care of God, as we understood Him. Critics like to jump all over this one because of the use of the word God and its religious implications. Let's be clear. The Step refers to God "as we understood him." This means that it is a subjective experience and it is that subjective nature that makes it spiritual by definition. Religion is formalized and presents fixed beliefs, traditions, and rituals. Spirituality, on the other hand, is a subjective experience. I had an Intensive Outpatient Program group go around and give me another word for God. They came up with "belief system, morality, consciousness, faith, awareness, inner beliefs, inner strength, support, meaning, care, never alone, help, hope, peace, love, dreams, happiness, compassion, joy, direction, guidance, power, serenity, wisdom, and courage." I think you get the idea. Turning our life and will over simply means doing the right thing, and no one can object to that. When a mistake is made, one does the next right thing and so forth. When we take the 3rd Step, this is what we are doing. But make no mistake, this is an action step. We actively make a decision based on our willingness and faith, and consciously hold onto this throughout the day (Alcoholics Anoymous, 2002; Narcotics Anonymous, 1984).

Step 4. We made a searching and fearless, moral inventory of ourselves. Hmm! Sounds daunting. People often have a harder time starting this than they do writing it. Moral means concerned with right and wrong behavior. If folks only knew what was in store for them! I don't mean sitting there hour after hour trying to write your life story. I mean experiencing the benefits of becoming cleared out and cleaned out. That's where this is going. The 4th Step helps the addict/alcoholic learn honesty and humility, eliminates the power the past has over them, and lays the groundwork for future Steps (Springborn, 1992). Step 4 helps the addict/alcoholic learn who they are (Alcoholics Anonymous, 2002; Narcotics Anonymous, 1984). There are many ways to approach a 4th step and no wrong way to accomplish it. There are many guides that offer direction. I recommend just starting with what is right in front of one's nose. What are the things that bother one most and why, and proceed in this fashion. Most people, given a little time to focus, can come up with a short list of what bothers them the most about themselves, their behavior, and their lives, pretty quickly. Some guides tell you to start with lists about people (mom, dad, wife, husband, etc.). Some guides have you make charts of feelings (resentment, anger, selfishness, etc). I say, keep it simple. If one is honest, careful, and thorough, one will come up with common denominators that relate to most of the troublesome things in your life. If there are things that have not been included, one can go back and enter it.

Step 5. We admitted to God, to ourselves, and another human being, the exact nature of our wrongs. That's right, you're going to share your 4th Step! The cleansing has begun! The addict/alcoholic has lived in isolation; Step 5 brings light to the dark corners of one's life (Alcoholics Anonymous, 2002; Narcotics Anonymous, 1984). This person should be selected carefully. It may be a sponsor, a clergy, a counselor, or a trusted friend. Some prefer clergy or professionals because they know these people are bound by confidentiality. One wants someone who can keep your confidentiality, who has an understanding of the Steps, who is mature and wise, and willing to share their own experiences (Spirngborn, 1992). The 'exact nature of our wrongs' must be shared, otherwise it will repeat itself if it is held onto inside (Alcoholics Anonymous, 2002; Narcotics Anonymous, 1984). Sharing the 4th Step often brings about disclosure on the part of the person one is sharing it with. The experience is exceedingly cathartic. Addiction is filled with secrets and isolation. Finally, one no longer has to carry that pervasive, encumbering, burden around every waking moment. He is free of it!

Step 6. We were entirely ready to have God remove these character defects. The cleansing process continues. Step 6 implies two things. First, looking at one's 4th Step, and with the help of a sponsor, coming up with a list of recurring themes. For example, if one's anger continues to create consequences as reflected in the 4th Step, anger may then be considered a "defect." If one's self-doubt and low-esteem continually crops up and interferes with one's functioning, then this, too, is a defect. I have always hated the word defect. It sounds like a tire factory reject. It is meant to point toward our deficiencies – areas in which we are lacking. We all have them. But Step 6 is tricky! First we have identified these 'defects.' Okay. And it stands to reason we would want them removed, right? Well, maybe and maybe not. There are two problems. First, we may be getting needs met by a particular defect. Maybe our anger really puts up a smokescreen for our insecurities. Take away the anger and one must not only be upfront about those inadequacies, but one must begin to deal with them. So it's not so simple. Then, we are supposed to be "entirely" ready to have them removed. Truth is, this is a process and in many cases, that's as close as we honestly get. We strive for willingness in this Step (Alcoholics Anonymous, 2002; Narcotics Anonymous, 1984). We may need to revisit Step 3 in order to remind ourselves that this is a good thing after all. In other words, we accepted that a Higher Power could restore order in our life and that turning our lives over is a good thing. We need to let go and trust. In Steps 1 and 2, we surrender our addiction; in Step 3 we surrender our will; and now in Step 6, we surrender once again because we see how our defects have fed our addiction (Springborn, 1992). Those patterns of behavior have become "hardwired" (p. 2). "Surrender is the seed of hope" (p. 3).

Step 7. We humbly asked him to remove our shortcomings. If we have done a good Step 6; then Step 7 comes easy. Again, Steps 6 and 7 are a continual process. We may never be completely relieved of a particular shortcoming, but we may reach more functional levels. If one's life has been ravaged by shame, and one has gone from an all-pervasive influence in life to fleeting recall, that is rather exceptional. By this time, we have begun a transformation. We have begun to feel a Higher Power working in our lives and can now turn once again with faith and humility. We have learned we are not "wrong;" we are human. This is the difference between humiliation, which is shame based and humility, which is understanding oneself in relationship to one's Higher Power. Our transformation is about finding strength in our weakness. In Step 7, we wish to be relieved of destructive aspects of our personalities (Alcoholics Anonymous, 2002; Narcotics Anonymous, 1984).

Step 8. We made a list of all persons we had harmed and became willing to make amends to them all. We can get our list from our 4th Step. Becoming willing to make amends does not just mean saying, "I'm sorry." Amends means to change; thus we must be willing to demonstrate new behavior so as not to inflict harm again. We are gaining a new understanding of ourselves and how to deal with other people (Alcoholics Anonymous, 2002; Narcotics Anonymous, 1984). This must be shown not said and Step 8 is preparing to "clean up our messes" (Spingborn, 1992, p. 3). But all we must do at this stage, is to become willing. In Step 3, we became willing to turn our life and will over; in Step 6, we became willing to remove our defects; now we become willing to make amends – a familiar process. People we have harmed also includes ourselves. We take Step 8 to become free of the guilt we have carried around so long, and continue to be cleaned out (Alcoholics Anonymous, 2002; Narcotics Anonymous, 1984).

Step 9. We made direct amends to such people wherever possible, except when to do so would injure them or others. Direct amends then means showing those persons, by our changes, that we have been intrinsically moved by our mistakes, not just sorry. They flared up back at us, and of course we are doing our utmost to prevent such influences from affecting other's lives again, and that we have an understanding that our actions say much more than our words. This is an action step and it need not be unpleasant (Springborn, 1992). Typically, we are relieved of shame, guilt, remorse, and fear. What does it mean by "except when to do so would injure them or others?" There are situations when it is better to "say nothing and let our changed behavior do the talking" (Springborn, 1992, p. 8)

Step 10. We continued to take personal inventory and when we were wrong, promptly admitted it. Best done on a daily and as needed basis. Once we have achieved serenity in our lives, we don't want to lose. We have learned that it is wise to take care of our problems and mistakes immediately as they arise. We have developed little tolerance for things that disturb our peace of mind. We are ready and waiting for Step 11. By continuing to do Step 10, we continue to be set free (Alcoholics Anonymous, 2002; Narcotics Anonymous, 1984).

Step 11. We sought through prayer and meditation to improve our consciousness with God as we understand him, praying only for knowledge of His will for us and the power to carry that out. We wish to perpetuate our newfound freedom. Prayer is talking with our Higher Power and meditation is listening (Alcoholics Anonymous, 2002; Narcotics Anonymous, 1984). We now have a partnership with our Higher Power (Springborn, 1992). We are learning to listen intuitively to what is the right thing, and the next right thing, to do. This is how we gain knowledge of His will for us and achieve the power to carry it out.

Step 12. Having had a spiritual awakening as a result of these steps, we tried to carry this message to alcoholics, and to practice these principles in all our affairs. Just as we learned in Step 1 that we had to lose ourself to find ourself; we learned in Step 12 that we must now give away what we have in order to keep it (Alcoholics Anonymous, 2002; Narcotics Anonymous, 1984). Furthermore, having found this way to work with our addiction, we practice what we've learned in all other areas of our lives. Our awakening has been a transformation to happiness, joyfulness, and freedom. We have been cleared out and cleaned out by this Step process. We sought a spiritual solution more powerful than our addiction (Springborn, 1992, p. 2). How did this happen? In Step 1, we said "I can't." In Step 2, we said, "God can." In Step 3, we said, "we will let Him." We cleaned house in Steps 4, 5, 6, 7, 8, and 9. And in Steps 10 and 11, we continued to maintain and connect with our Higher Power. Now in Step 12, we put our faith into action. This awakening is so much more than we could have come up with on our own terms. We have learned that things we did not think were possible – are possible. And we take joy in imparting this to others.

SPIRITUALITY AND RELIGION

Some people find recovery through spirituality and/or religion separate and distinct from AA. Today, there is much research that supports a positive relationship with spirituality and wellness (Miller & Thoresen, 2003). Spirituality has been correlated with a higher quality of life (Galanter, 2005; Temple University, 2009; Han, 2009; Liberman, 2008; Heintzman, 2008; Delgado, 2007). Miller and Thoreson (2003) suggest this is an area requiring more research. In dual-diagnosis treatment today, spirituality is often presented topically and minimally as a coping strategy in treatment. However, in 2006 the Substance Abuse and Mental Health Service Administration (SAMHSA), a division of the U.S. Department of Health and Human Services, which sets policy and direction for government-subsidized agencies, published principles for effective integrated care. Principle 10 states "Treatment should be individualized to accommodate the specific needs, personal goals, and cultural perspectives of unique individuals in different stages of change." This principle embraces the inclusion of religiosity/spirituality (R/S). Many clients desire it (Koenig, 2007). Fallot (1998) states that the inclusion of R/S is a holistically and culturally competent approach and can be included in recovery plans (formally treatment goals) identifying problems, goals, and resources. Spiritual goals may include gaining hope and meaning; strengthening a relationship with what is referred to as a transcendent; i.e., God or a Higher Power; perseverance; resolving anger; frustration or disappointment; forgiveness; gaining a sense of guidance; and understanding why God allows bad things to happen (Huguelet & Koenig, 2009).

Because spirituality has been demonstrated to be instrumental for a sense of well-being (Miller & Thoreson, 2003), it is useful to study how dual-diagnosed clients achieve spirituality to better inform and train practitioners to include this aspect of recovery in treatment modalities. R/S is beginning to be incorporated in treatment in a variety of ways. McKinney (2009) supports partnering with the R/S community as an effective strategy. R/S may become the 4th dimension in the bio-psycho-social evaluation (Huguelet & Koenig, 2009). Examples include the Matrix System (Ramson, 2005) and Pathways to Recovery (Ridgway et al., 2002). Both introduce the R/S topic in a workbook-style approach. Both are designed to get the client thinking in the R/S direction and what their perspective is (what R/S means to them, how they define it, what their role with R/S may be, obstacles in R/S, and how, if right for them, they may incorporate R/S into their lives). There are also faith-based programs which have more of an emphasis on R/S than CBT (Huguelet & Koenig, 2009). There are several focuses of such programs including: fostering tolerance, self-awareness, exploration of values, enhancing recovery, providing new information on R/S, forgiveness, moving from victimization to resilience, and the usage of R/S tapes and resources to develop strength and hope.

Due to the fact that dual-diagnosed persons face significant obstacles and suffer poor quality of life, it is necessary to include R/S in treatment programs as it is one means that has been associated with wellness (Gail et al., 2005; Gail, 2003; Cohen, 2002; Gordon et al., 2002; Delgado, 2007). Furthermore, understanding the development of spiritual components, which may enhance and/or become the foundation of recovery, the focus of this proposed study is imperative.

Spirituality has been a controversial topic to address in substance abuse facilities. It is typically found in 12-Step Programs, such as Alcoholics Anonymous. Initially, there appeared to be an assumption that spirituality (a) could not be studied scientifically and (b) should not be studied scientifically. Today, though, there is much research that supports a positive relationship with spirituality and wellness (Miller & Thoresen, 2003).

According to the Connecticut Department of Mental Health and Addiction Services (DMHAS), which has adopted the national Substance Abuse and Mental Health Administration's (SAMHSA) proposed model of recovery and recovery-oriented services, IDDT has several basic recovery premises. These were reviewed in Chapter 15, but for our purposes in this unit, treatment must be approached holistically and programming must be flexible to incorporate individual recovery plans.

IDDT Recovery Dimensions include understanding how behaviors affect recovery; hope, confidence, and commitment; understanding and accepting oneself; relationships with family, friends, and supportive others; maintaining recovery; supports in the community to enhance recovery; promoting recovery, and becoming an empowered citizen.

While the objectives of these Recovery Core Values are clear about dealing with the client as an individual in a strengths-based fashion and a collaborative manner, the aspect of spirituality counseling in treatment programs is controversial. It is another example of standards and practices not meeting up with goals and aspirations.

In treatment today, spirituality is either dealt with briefly as solutions-focused strategy, referred out, or simply not included at all. In addition, cognitive-behavioral therapy is also employed in the form of psycho-education and more directive therapy. The Matrix System, for example, includes coverage of a number of topics, which are considered to be triggers for the substance abuser, along with the provision of related coping strategies and skills (Ramson, Obert, McCann, & Ling, 2005). Triggers include, but are not limited to: work, money, boredom, relationships, anger, friends and family, cravings, mental illness, loneliness, hunger, tiredness, and so forth (Ramson, Obert, McCann, & Ling, 2005). CBT techniques offer specific solutions-focused responses, methods, and inclusion of individualized spiritual practices (Ramson, Obert, McCann, & Ling, 2005). Thus, spirituality practices are acknowledged and included as part of Cognitve Behavioral Therapy. These techniques parallel what is referred to as positive psychology, that is, methods that can enhance happiness and actualizing.

Another example of this is Pathways to Recovery (Ridgway et al., 2002), which is mentioned earlier. It introduces the R/S topic in a workbook-style approach. It is designed to get the client thinking in the R/S direction and what their perspective is (what R/S means to them, how they define it, what their role with R/S may be, obstacles in R/S, and how, if right for them, may they incorporate R/S into their lives).

There are also faith-based programs, which have more of an emphasis on R/S than CBT (Huguelet & Koenig, 2009). There are several focuses of such programs including: fostering tolerance, self-awareness, exploration of values, enhancing recovery, providing new information on R/S, forgiveness, moving from victimization to resilience, and the usage of R/S tapes and resources to develop strength and hope As discussed, Huguelet and Koenig (2009) distinguish between spirituality and religiosity in a way that provides a distinction between the two concepts. Accordingly, religion is considered to indicate "specific behavioral, social, doctrinal, and denominational characteristics" (p. 1). It includes the notion of a transcendent in a ritualistic and formalized manner. Spirituality is concerned with "ultimate questions of life's meaning" (p.1) in a subjective way. The term spirituality eludes specific operational definitions. It is likely to differ when individuals speak of the spiritual, though it is generally referring to the non-material. It may or may not include religion. It often, however, may fall into four areas: a person's relationship with God; the deepest level from which a human being operates; the philosophical context of a person's life, including values, rules, attitudes and views; the same as religion. Huguelet and Koenig (2009) review four programs that integrate R/S issues with mental health by integrating CBT groups with R/S, R/S issue discussion groups, and integrating spiritual counseling with psychotherapy. Based on a client survey, these approaches were associated with positive outcomes.

Miller and Thoreson (2003) cite studies (Gallup, 2003) that demonstrate that 95% of the population has a belief in God. They cite numerous studies (Cole & Pargament, 1999; Dein & Stygal, 1997; Koenig, 1997; Pargament, 1997; Pargament, Smith, Koenig, & Perez, 1998) that have shown that spirituality can have an important influence on health and behavior. There have been assumptions that spirituality could not and should not be the subject of research (Miller & Thoreson, 2003). Furthermore, it may be useful to distinguish spirituality from religion. Miller and Thoreson (2003) state that the area of spirituality is in need of further research. Kendler et al., (2003) researched how spirituality and religion help to shield the distressing effects of life events and may relieve anxiety and depression. In a survey of 2,616 men and women, a 78-item questionnaire assessed various aspects of broadly defined spiritual/religious topics, which were found to have a positive effect on major depression, generalized anxiety disorder, phobias, panic disorder, and substance abuse. The results do not address the nature by which individuals with co-occurring disorders approach and address spirituality. Gallanter (2006) documents the spiritual aspects found in Alcoholics Anonymous and their adaptations to treatment facilities. He cites studies (Goldfarb et al., 1996; Molpovich et al., 1996) in which dual-diagnosed clients ranked the importance of spirituality higher than social service support and outpatient treatment. Gallanter et al (2007), in a self-rated scale, which reflected a broad view spiritual orientation to life, dual-diagnosed clients indicated that spirituality was an important aspect of their recovery. The importance of this was that it indicated that the relevance of spirituality is underestimated in the approach of treatment facilities.

Spirituality has been defined by Miller and Thoreson (2003) citing William James as the "feelings, acts, and experiences of individual men [sic] in their solitude . . . in relation to whatever they may consider the divine." The Oxford English Dictionary discusses two themes. The first is regarding life's most vital quality as giving life and energy to human elements of the person. Second, spirituality is a broad focus, including immaterial features of life regarded as imperceptible by the human senses. Spiritual terminology includes that which is transcendental, sacred, holy, or divine. The concept is multidimensional and spiritual practices may include relationships with others and/or a transcendent relationship. The concept does not have boundaries (Miller & Thoreson, 2003). The term spirituality eludes specific operational definitions. It is likely to differ when individuals speak of the spiritual, though it is generally referring to the non-material. It may or may not include religion. It often, however, may fall into four areas: a person's relationship with God; the deepest level from which a human being operates; the philosophical context of a person's life, including values, rules, attitudes and views; and for some, it may be the same as religion. However, if there is a distinction between spirituality and religion, it is that religion is usually formalized and institutionalized.

According to McCormick (2004) one of the earliest studies into spirituality was Francis Galton in 1869 in a paper called "Statistical Inquiries Into the Efficacy of Prayer." Other early studies include Durkheim's (1897-1951) theories of spirituality as a motivating force and William James' The Varieties of Religious Experience (1902) – just a historical footnote here.

Americans are very involved with spirituality in their lives. Koenig (2008) reports that 93% believe in God and 89% report belonging to a religious organization. Anandarajah (2001) reports that 77% of Americans think their doctors should consider their religious needs – 66% want their doctors to talk about spirituality if they were to be gravely ill and 10-20% state that their doctors do discuss spirituality. In other words, most people want spirituality included in their lives.

Huguelet and Koenig (2009) distinguish between spirituality and religiosity in a way that provides a distinction between the two concepts. Accordingly, religion is considered to indicate "specific behavioral, social, doctrinal, and denominational characteristics" (p. 1). It includes the notion of a transcendent in a ritualistic and formalized manner. Spirituality is concerned with "ultimate questions of life's meaning" (p. 1) in a subjective way.

Thus, there are certainly spiritual elements when defining religion; i.e., a transcendent construct. However, religion is typically formalized. Spirituality may include religiosity, but not necessarily. It tends to be a more subjective process. The terms are not interchangeable. The suggestion in this book is that clients be shown how to employ spirituality into their recovery (which may or may not include 'God' or religion. Much of the research cited is concerned with both religiosity and spirituality and do not necessarily make a distinction.

Spirituality and wellness. Gail et al., (2005) surmise that an increase in research into spirituality may be due to the fact that many people look to spiritual principles in times of need. They have developed a spiritual framework of coping. Often, people look to find cause in regard to illness or tragedy in order to make sense of it (Gail, 2003). This is called causal attribution and accounts for the foundation of this framework; spiritual appraisal. (Gail et al., 2005). Next, personal factors come into play; i.e., denomination or individual doctrine, problem-solving methods, and the inclusion of hope. People utilize behaviors involved with spiritual coping, including traditional and non-traditional spiritual practices. Spiritual coping may be a response to frequent stress (Gail et al., 2005). This may include prayer as a means of connectedness (Gail et al., 2005). Connectedness is the next step in the spiritual framework and may take different forms; i.e., nature, family and religious/spiritual communities, and/or a relationship with a Higher Power or God (Gail et al., 2005). Studies show that religion/spirituality play an important part for people in making meaning of life (Cohen, 2002; Gordon et al., 2002). This spiritual framework for appraisal, attribution, personal coping factors, connectedness, and meaning in life may come together toward emotional, social, physical, and spiritual well-being (Gail et al., 2005). Gail et al., (2005) suggest more research is needed to study the "pathways of effects" (p.97) for spiritual factors; in other words, how spirituality works to enhance coping and well-being.

Delgado (2007) investigated the correlation between a sense of coherence and perceived level of stress, quality of life, and spirituality in those with chronic illnesses. Results indicated that spirituality may buffer stress for those chronically ill. One drawback from the study was that over 90% of those tested were Caucasian which may tend to skew results.

O'Connel and Skevington (2005) measured quality of life, spirituality, religion, and personal beliefs in adult focus groups. Spiritual strength was among the most important. The results improve the case for a biopsychosocial-spiritual model of health. The average age of participants was 51 and raises the question regarding younger people. The groups were also biased by a predominance of well-educated participants.

Hill and Pargament (2008) ask why is it that religion/spirituality are correlated with health? They suggest the answer lies in the nature of religion/spirituality. Initially, they distinguish between religion and spirituality by defining religion as a "fixed system of ideas or ideological commitments" (p. 3) and spirituality as an "individual, subjective, emotional, inward, unsystematic, freeing expression" (p. 3). Furthermore, Hill and Pargament (2008) state there is somewhat of a polarization of religion and spirituality. Hill and Hood (1999) indicate religion and spirituality are not uniform processes but complex variables. Both spirituality and religion can be orienting and motivating forces and both may use perceived closeness to God as the ultimate value (Hill & Pargament, 2008). Expanding on this discussion would allow you to address my earlier comments about defining religion and spirituality, and how you will be exploring one or both in the study. This study is ultimately interested in the dual-diagnosed recovering person's growth that allows them to live in sobriety and achieve a high quality of life. As spoken in the rooms of Alcoholics Anonymous, what is it that allows the member to live in a "happy, joyous, and free" manner? This expression is typically used when describing life after working the 12 Steps of AA. The 12 Steps of AA, of course, represent a spiritual program. That growth of the recovering dual-diagnosed individual, typically involves a "power greater than themselves" (Step 3). That "power" need not be a transcendent. It is not the type of Higher Power that is important, but the notion of human limitations and a power greater than ourselves (Riordan & Walsh, 1994). For many, that power is within the self; a 'bigger' self that is attuned to higher values and meaning in life, rather than the 'small self' one was accustomed to. This line of thought does not require individuals to look outside themselves if that is problematic (Davis, Golie, & Jansen, 1998). For some, this growth may include religion.

Based on compilations of research studies, religiosity and spirituality are correlated to lower blood pressure, less hypertension, better lipid profiles, and better immune function (Seeman, Dubin, & Seeman, 2003). Zen, yoga, meditation/relaxation processes are associated with lower blood pressure, lower cholesterol, less oxidative stress, and better health outcomes in clinical patients (Seeman, Dubin, & Seeman, 2003).

Spirituality and dual-diagnosis treatment. In 2006, SAMSHA published principles of effective integrated care. Principle 10 states, "Treatment should be individualized to accommodate the specific needs, personal goals, and cultural perspectives of unique individuals in different stages of change." The Department of Mental Health and Addiction Services (DMHAS) defines recovery as such: "The Department endorses a broad vision of recovery that involves a process of restoring or developing a positive sense of identity and meaningful sense of belonging apart from one's condition, and then rebuilding a life despite or within the limitations imposed by that condition. A recovery-oriented system of care identifies and builds upon each person's assets, strengths, and areas of health and competence to support the person in managing his or her condition while regaining a meaningful, constructive sense of membership in the broader community."

These principles embrace the inclusion of religiosity and/or spirituality (R/S) for many reasons. Koenig (2007) states that R/S is a part of many clients' lives and many would like it to be addressed. R/S influences the client's ability to cope. When hospitalized, clients are removed from the R/S community. R/S is associated with mental and physical health. Fallot (1998) states that the inclusion of R/S is a holistically and culturally competent approach and can be included in recovery plans (formally treatment goals) identifying problems, goals, and resources. Spiritual goals may include gaining hope and meaning; strengthening a relationship with what is referred to as a transcendent; i.e., God, or a Higher Power; perseverance; resolving anger; frustration or disappointment; forgiveness; understanding why God allows bad things to happen; and gaining a sense of guidance (Huguelet & Koenig, 2009). In a qualitative study involving the R/S experiences of mental health clients, Fallot (1998) identifies several dimensions emerging from the narratives. They include: whole-person involvement; recovery as a long-term journey; hope as an essential ingredient; importance of divine love as strengthening and sustaining; the inclusion of the serenity prayer in order to cope; developing authenticity; i.e., finding one's True Self; and centering; action; pragmatism; and conviction. Sullivan (1998) identified several factors contributing to recovery as derived by a survey of mental health clients. They include medication, vocational assistance, family and friends, coping and decision-making skills, social support, coherence, and 43% indicated spirituality.

The next question then is how to include spirituality in treatment programs? Koenig (2007) suggests R/S can be included in the screening process. This involves listening to understand, showing respect, supporting beliefs, and an appropriate referral (Koenig, 2007). McKinney et al., (2009) supports partnering with the R/S community as an effective strategy. R/S may become the 4th dimension in the bio-psycho-social evaluation (Huguelet & Koenig, 2009). Rose, Westefeld, and Ansely (2001) state that many psychologists have little training in religious/spiritual issues, and using a survey did a study to assess the appropriateness of clinicians discussing religious/

spiritual issues. There is some evidence suggesting clients would like their therapist to talk about these issues. Data suggests many prefer clinicians who have beliefs similar to their own. Some clients have concerns that the counselor may alter or undermine their beliefs, and believe that those in secular positions may be less sensitive. Huguelet and Koenig (2009) suggest that psycho-educational cognitive-behavioral therapy (CBT) groups can be enhanced with the inclusion of spiritual frameworks.

Huguelet and Koenig (2009) review four programs that integrate R/S issues with mental health by integrating CBT groups with R/S, R/S issue discussion groups, and integrating spiritual counseling with psychotherapy. Based on a client survey, these approaches were associated with positive outcomes. Piedmont (2004) researched spirituality in relation to substance abuse treatment programs. Spirituality is defined as a personal attribute, like a personality construct and religion encompassing beliefs and practices of an institutional nature. While positive outcomes have been associated with AA, substance abuse programs, and spirituality, none researched the predictive effects of spirituality on treatment. Piedmont (2004) used a Spiritual Transcendence Scale to measure three facets of spirituality: prayer fulfillment, universality, and connectedness, which were positively correlated with positive treatment outcomes. Piedmont (2004) suggests further research is needed to assess the spiritual qualities of clients.

There can be negative results including R/S in treatment as well (Koenig, 2007; Hugeulet & Koenig, 2009). Some clients may not find the inclusion of R/S helpful and may actually find it harmful because contemplating the topic may be a burden.They may be angry with God, question the existence of a transcendent, or may be disconcerted with the R/S community (Hugeulet & Koenig, 2009). The mental health/substance abuse counselor may be untrained in R/S matters (Koenig, 2007). Some clients have harmful experiences with R/S, such as finding R/S involvement judgmental and/or alienating, and there may be inner struggles creating conflict. There may be trying values; i.e., sexual morality, honesty, generosity, forgiveness which generates guilt, self-condemnation, and discouragement (Koenig, 2007).

PSYCHOTHERAPY, SOLUTIONS-FOCUSED THERAPY, MEDICATIONS

Three more methods of recovery are psychotherapy, cognitive behavioral therapy- based solutions-focused treatment, and the use of medications.

Not all clients coming in for substance use treatment meet the criteria for chemical dependency. There are many who land in treatment as a result of crisis. There are two types of crisis: conflict and situational. A situational crisis is a temporary situation; i.e, divorce, loss of a loved one, or job loss. Once resolved, the crisis is over, as are the symptomatic fallout – which in this case may be substance use. A crisis rising out of conflict implies a long-term, unresolved issue; perhaps abandonment, abuse, loss, a traumatic incident, and so forth. All of these are examples of clients who may benefit from psychotherapy (interpretative oriented) or counseling (skills oriented) for a brief or even long-term period. Issues can reach a state of sufficient resolution that they no longer impact on the client in a pervasive or critical manner.

Solutions-focused treatment is cognitive-behavioral therapy in the form of psycho-education and more directive therapy. The Matrix System, for example, includes coverage of a number of topics, which are considered to be triggers for the substance abuser along with the provision of related coping strategies and skills (Ramson, Obert, McCann, & Ling, 2005). Triggers include, but are not limited to: work, money, boredom, relationships, anger, friends and family, cravings, mental illness, loneliness, hunger, tiredness, and so forth

(Ramson, Obert, McCann, & Ling, 2005). In addition, Rational Emotive Therapy is used. RET looks at a set of circumstances and creates a formula where "A" is the environmental event that the individual is presented with, "B" is the thought they have in response to "A", and "C" is the emotional behavior they have in response to "B." The theory is that our behavior is based on our thinking – not an external event. The counselor tries to help the client alter irrational ideas they have in response to events, thereby changing their behavior – in this case, substance. Some people respond to these successfully and are able to change their behavior by employing these new coping strategies.

Lastly, there are those with a co-occurring disorder; i.e., anxiety or depression, who respond very well to medication and have a "medication awakening," if you will. Basically, sometimes, the addition of a medication addresses the primary motivation for substance usage and the client no longer chooses to self-medicate.

> *Comment for the Reader:* The 12-Step process, religion and spirituality, solutions-focusing, psychotherapy, and medication management all have one common denominator. Have you figured it out? Change. They all imply major change in the way people think, feel, and behave. I love it. Like they say in the rooms, "If nothing changes, nothing changes!"

CHAPTER 27

STAGES OF SPIRITUALITY

This writer recently conducted an exploratory research study to understand the essence of recovering (5+ years) dual-diagnosed individuals' experiences with spirituality. By the essence of their experiences, the study sought to understand the development, motivation, driving forces, dynamics, mechanics and maintenance, of their spirituality.

Why? First of all, addressing co-occurring disorders in counseling has become primordial. Co-occurring disorders is now the rule, not the exception. Also, those with dual diagnoses often face greater obstacles than those with primary mental health disorders and experience higher relapse frequency and poorer quality of life. Furthermore, spirituality is closely correlated with increased quality of life. So it only made sense to me to better understand how spirituality works in the lives of those with dual diagnoses.

RESEARCH DESIGN STRATEGY

Qualitative phenomenological study is a reflective process regarding people's every- day experiences (Crotty, 1998). There is an effort on the part of the researcher to put themself in the place of the other (Crotty, 1998). The individual's experience, perceptions and meaning are emphasized. The intent is to describe from the point of view of the participant. The subjective experience is what distinguishes it from other qualitative research. It is about how the participants experience life around them and interpret the world, in this case spirituality. Conversational analysis is at the core of this form of qualitative study. It is an effort to focus inquiry on the meanings and values of the participants (Crotty, 1998).

Unstructured 90-minute interviews were used with seven participants. The interviews were audiotaped. Content analysis used an interpretative approach. This means that units of meaning and levels of meaning were analyzed from the interview conversational text. The use of concepts and semantics predominated. Data was then be interpreted and elaborated on regarding its content.

Sampling Design

The population at large is all dual-diagnosed persons in recovery for five years or more in the U.S. with a strong sense of spirituality. The sample was a convenience and purposive one. This means that participants, who met the study's requirements, were selected based on facility. The age range in this proposed study from 30 to 70 and consisted of both men and women. Persons known to the researcher was from local AA meetings were asked to be participants. It is a convenience sample because participants will be in close proximity to where the researcher lives in northwestern CT. It is a purposive sample because participants will be selected based on being 5+ years in recovery, having both a substance abuse and another mental health diagnosis, and having a strong sense of spirituality. Some participants may still be involved in outpatient mental health counseling; others may not. The AA groups are not affiliated with any behavioral health organization. Furthermore, it is stated in the 12 Traditions of AA that each group is autonomous, there is not a governing body, and is not organized. Instead, there are service boards when it comes to matters affecting other groups or AA as a whole. Therefore, this researcher was able to ask persons that he knew to participate in the study without formalized approval. Participants were recruited from known contacts within the Farmington Valley of CT who are involved in AA or NA.

MEASURES

In qualitative phenomenological studies, the researcher is the instrument collecting data through a process of unstandardized interviews aimed at discovering, understanding, and interpreting the essence of experiences as described by participants regarding their spiritual development. (Kostere, 2006). Semi-structured interview questions were used as guidelines (Berg, 2007).

Interview Questions:

1) What was your drug of choice?
2) How long did you use for?
3) How did you get into recovery?
4) How long have you been in recovery?
5) Did you relapse?
6) What is your mental health diagnosis?
7) How was this diagnosed?
8) Are you or have you been on medications?
9) Tell me your story.
10) How did your substance abuse impact on your mental illness?
11) How did your mental illness impact on your substance abuse?
12) What does spirituality mean to you?

    For example;

    A person's relationship with a higher power

    The deepest level from which a human being operates

    The philosophical context of a person's life (values, rules, attitudes, and views)

    The same as religion

13) When did you first have a sense of spirituality?
14) How did spirituality develop for you?
15) What steps were involved?
16) How does spirituality affect your recovery?
17) Did your dual diagnosis affect your spirituality?
18) Is there a relationship between your recovery and spirituality?

This study included a heuristic component, which means it includes the personal experience and insight of the researcher (Patton, 2002).

Data Collection Procedures

The researcher attended local AA meetings and identified prospective participants by informing known members that he was looking for volunteers to participate in a research study regarding the spiritual development and experiences of dual-diagnosed individuals: the criteria is that individuals have a dual diagnosis, 5 plus years of recovery, and who consider themselves to have a strong sense of spirituality. The participants were asked to sign informed consents and appointments for 90-minute interviews will be scheduled. The interviews were conducted and a phenomenological model was utilized. There are two processes involved in the phenomenological model that were used in this proposed study (Kostere, Kostere, & Percy, 2008).

1) Interviews were conducted and original data was obtained comprised of descriptions from open-ended questions and dialogue.
2) The participants' accounts and experiences were structured based on reflective analysis and interpreted by the researcher.

DATA ANALYSIS PROCEDURES

Following the interviews and transcription, the data was analyzed and interpreted. Through the epoche process of phenomenological reduction, the researcher identified his prior knowledge and experience of the subject, and intentionally put it aside in order that the data from the research may speak for itself. The researcher consciously remained open to what revealed itself and assumed nothing (Giorgi, 1997).

Giorgi (1997) describes a 5-Step model to organizing and describing the data that shall be followed in this proposed study.

1) The interviews were transcribed into written form. This researcher used Dragon Macspeech “Dictate” software, which transcribed voice-to-text onto a document format.
2) The researcher read all the data and got a sense of the whole.
3) The researcher discriminated the data into ‘meaning units’ and identified clusters of themes which were restricted or combined into manageable and understandable concepts.
4) The researcher then synthesized the themes taking everyday expressions, and transformed them into psychological language with an emphasis on the research subject matter, and created a composite of the experiences of the participants.

LIMITATIONS OF RESEARCH DESIGN

The research methodology used for this proposed study is an interpretive qualitative in-depth interview approach. It is being completed in a middle to upper middle class suburban community in northwestern Connecticut. The study does not reflect lower socioeconomic opinions, attitudes, or accounts of experiences. Nor is its representation multi-cultural.

In order to ensure accuracy and credibility, there are several actions that were taken. The researcher was concerned whether the research uncovers what it sets out to do; basically, the spiritual experiences (spiritual development, relationship with a higher power, and so forth) of dual-diagnosed clients. The study results needed to mirror reality and there were several things that helped in this process.

First, the results were reviewed with the participants for accuracy, to compare interpretations for agreement and comment. Increased credibility can make for increased dependability. Second, colleagues were called upon to comment on the results. Third, 'thick' description of the interviews were used so that the reader can also draw their own conclusions. Lastly, the researcher's assumptions of philosophical and theoretical framework for the research were examined in detail as well as identifying what the study does not do. For example, the study hopefully provided data for further empirical quantitative research in order to possibly modify treatment planning and programs.

Results

First, although the scope of this study was confined to understanding the recovering dual-diagnosed individuals' spiritual experiences, it is necessary to mention that three themes emerged from the interviews, which seemed to be contained in the participants' accounts and experiences outside the focus of the research. In telling their story and explaining the role that spirituality plays in their lives, it was necessary to provide a background leading up to their multiple years in recovery as dual-diagnosed individuals.

The first theme detailed in all of the accounts was the nature of being 'out of control' with their addiction(s) and other mental health issues. The second theme demonstrated in all of the accounts was the nature of how substance abuse exacerbated their mental health issues and vice versa. Both of these have been the subjects of previous research. The third theme is that many of the accounts included the notion of 'self-medicating' their mental health issues via their substance usage. This is not a new concept either, and the researcher has seen more and more of this over the years as the dual-diagnosis paradigm has become accepted. These observations are certainly noteworthy, but are only indirectly related to the scope of this research.

After an analysis of the data, three areas of study emerged into categories: 1) motives for including spirituality in one's life, 2) how the spirituality developed, and 3) the maintenance and fulfillment derived from spirituality in their lives.

Within the first theme to emerge from the data was motives for the inclusion of spirituality in the participants' lives. In other words, there needed to be a basis for spirituality to be a part of their lives.

These motives fell into three categories:

1) Spirituality may have pre-existed in their lives prior to recovery. For example, it may have been part of their upbringing.
2) Spirituality may be the result of a profound experience that the participant considered to be spiritual in nature. For example, seeing an angel.
3) Spirituality is the result of having been 'broken' as an individual. For example, being in a state of desperation as a result of a series of events in their lives.

The second theme was spiritual development. This took two forms:

1) Involvement in the recovery process. In other words, achieving spiritual development by attending meetings; associating with others in recovery; 'working' the Steps, doing service work, being involved with sponsors and sponsees, and so forth.
2) Growth as a result of other spiritual pursuits such as religion, education, searching for enlightenment, and so forth.

The third theme was that of spiritual practices which fell into two categories:

1) Things people did to maintain their spirituality, such as reading meditation books, meditating, prayer, continue to work the steps, applying spiritual principles in all areas of their lives.
2) Fulfillment derived from spirituality. For example, becoming comfortable in their own skin, improved self-esteem, happiness, joyfulness, sensing freedom, relief from anxiety and depression, and so forth.

Having now completed a detailed analysis of the results of the data, a synthesization of the research transforms that product into pragmatic terms. The themes of 1) a spiritual basis [pre-existing, epiphany, and fatality] 2) spiritual development [recovery process, growth due to other means] and 3) spiritual practices [maintenance methods, resulting fulfillment] are viewed as *stages* of spirituality experienced by the recovering dual-diagnosed individuals participating in the study.

Viewing the presented themes as *stages in a process that support spiritual fulfillment* provides a composite of the experiences of the participants. Initially, the first stage includes the basis or origin for the presence of spirituality. The research demonstrated that people either had the seed planted as a child, experienced a profound revelation or epiphany, or were driven by desperation to seek out help from sources greater than themselves – or some combination thereof. The second stage involves spiritual development. The research demonstrated this may have come from the recovery process illustrated by AA/12-Step Program, which may include, but not limited to, attending meetings, associating with other recovering people in fellowship, 'working' the Steps, doing service work, and working with sponsors and sponsees. Spiritual development may have also come from growth in other areas, including, but not limited to, religion, education, prayer, meditation, being of service to others, and a relationship with a Higher Power. The third stage of the process includes practices that maintain one's spirituality and the experience of living a life endowed with spiritual fulfillment.

Recommendations

The long-range motivation of the researcher in conducting this study is the eventual inclusion of more comprehensive spirituality counseling within treatment programs. Further research may be needed in at least two areas.

Conclusion

Jnit 7 has reviewed working the 12 Steps, inclusion gion into recovery, utilizing psychotherapy and/or medications, as well as focusing on skills and strategies – they are all methods that may be employed in recovering from co-occurring disorders. Our discussion of Stages of Spirituality provides information that can be utilized to enhance the client's spiritual growth.

UNIT 7 Highlights

CH 26: Five Ways to Recover

- 12-Step Process/cleaning out process/brings about psychic change
- Religiosity/fixed and formal belief system
- Spirituality/subjective belief system
- Religion/spirituality correlated with wellness and increased quality of life
- Psychotherapy/conflict resolution
- CBT/coping and skill strategies address triggers to use
- Medications/address chemical imbalance, psychiatric illness/"medication awakening"

CH 27: Stages of spirituality

- Basis for spirituality = pre-existing/revelation/broken-ness
- Spiritual development = the recovery process/searching for enlightenment
- Spiritual practices = maintenance/fulfillment

STUDY GUIDE

1) What are various means of recovering from addiction/alcoholism?
2) What is the essential ingredient of Recovery methods?
3) Why is it important to understand stages of spirituality?

REFERENCES

Alcoholics Anonymous (1939). *Alcoholics Anonymous.* Alcoholics Anonymous World Services.

Andres-Hyman, R. (2004, December). *Recovery Core Values.* Handout Presented at Connecticut Department of Mental Health and Addiction Services Education and Training, Hartford, CT.

Cohen, A. (2002). The importance of spirituality in well-being for Jews and Christians. *Journal of Happiness Studies,* 3(3), 287-310. doi:10.1023/A:1020656823365.

Cole, B. & Pargament, K. (1999). Spiritual surrender: A paradoxical path to control. Integrating spirituality into treatment: Resources for practitioners (pp. 179-198). Washington, DC US: American Psychological Association. doi:10.1037/10327-009.

Davis, Diane Rae, and Golie G. Jansen (1998). "Making meaning of Alcoholics Anonymous for social workers: Myths, metaphors, and realities." *Social Work* 43(2), 169-182. PsycINFO, EBSCOhost (accessed December 12, 2009).

Delgado, C. (2007). Sense of Coherence, Spirituality, Stress and Quality of Life in Chronic Illness. *Journal of Nursing Scholarship,* 39(3), 229-34. Retrieved April 18, 2009, from ProQuest Psychology Journals database. (Document ID: 1428124701),

Fallot, R. (1998). *Spirituality and religion in recovery from mental illness.* New Directions of Mental Health Services. Los Angeles: Josey-Bass Publishers.

Galanter. M. (2008). Spirituality, Evidence-Based Medicine, and Alcoholics Anonymous. *The American Journal of Psychiatry,* 165(12), 1514-7. Retrieved April 18, 2009, from ProQuest Psychology Journals database. (Document ID: 1607951671).

Gordon, C. (2002, May). Women's stories: Spiritual journeys to herself. Dissertation Abstracts International Section A, 62, Retrieved from PsycINFO database.

Gall, T.; Charbonneau, C.; Clarke, N.; Grant, K.; Joseph, A.; & Shouldice, L. (2005). Understanding the Nature and Role of Spirituality in Relation to Coping and Health: A Conceptual Framework. *Canadian Psychology/Psychologiecanadienne.*

Goldfarb, L.; Galanter, M.; McDowell, D.; Lifshutz, H.; & Dermatis, H. (1996). Medical student and patient attitudes toward religion and spirituality in the recovery process. The American Journal of Drug and Alcohol Abuse, 22(4), 549-561. doi:10.3109/00952999609001680.

Han, J. (2008). Loneliness, spirituality, and depression in homebound older adults. *The Gerontologist: 61st Annual Scientific Meeting "Resilience in an Aging. SPECIAL ISSUE III*, 48, 620. Retrieved April 18, 2009, from ProQuest Psychology Journals database. (Document ID: 1647961601).

Hill, P. & Hood, R. (1999). Affect, religion and unconscious processes. Journal of Personality, 67(6), 1015-1046. doi:10.1111/1467-6494.00081.

Heintzman, P. (2008). Leisure-spiritual coping: A model for therapeutic recreation and leisure services. Therapeutic Recreation Journal, 42(1), 56-73. Retrieved from PsycINFO database.

Hill, P. & Pargament, K. (2003). Advances in the conceptualization and measurement of religion and spirituality: Implications for physical and mental health research. American Psychologist, 58(1), 64-74. doi:10.1037/0003-066X.58.1.64.

Hugeulet, P. & Koenig, H.G. (2009). Religion and spirituality in psychiatry. New York: Cambridge University Press.

Koenig, H.G. (2007). *Spirituality in patient care.* Conshohocken, PA: Templeton Press.

Liberman, R.P. (2008). Principles and Practice of Psychiatric Rehabilitation: An Empirical Approach. *The American Journal of Psychiatry,* 165(7), 924-925. Retrieved April 18, 2009, from ProQuest Psychology Journals database. (Document ID: 1508355881).

McCormick, D. (2004). Galton on Spirituality, Religion, and Health. *American Psychologist,* 59(1), 52. doi:10.1037/0003-066X.59.1.52a.

McKinney, S. (2009). Faith and spirituality in recovery. A Handout in a Presentation by the Connecticut Department of Mental Health and Addiction Services, Middletown, Connecticut.

Miller, W. & Thoresen, C. (2003, January). Spirituality, religion, and health: An emerging research field. *American Psychologist,* 58(1), 24-35. Retrieved April 7, 2009, doi:10.1037/0003-066X.58.1.24.

Narcotics Anonymous (6th ed.) (2008). NY. World Service office.

O'Connell, K.A.; Skevington, S.M. (2005). The relevance of spirituality, religion, and personal beliefs to health-related quality of life: Themes from focus groups in Britain. *British Journal of Health Psychology,* 3-10, 379-98.

Pargament, K. (1997). The psychology of religion and coping: Theory, research, practice. New York, NY. US: Guilford Press. Retrieved from PsycINFO database.

Pargament, K.; Smith, B.; Koenig, H.; & Perez, L. (1998). Patterns of positive and negative religious coping with major life stressors. Journal for the Scientific Study of Religion, 37(4), 710-724. doi:10.2307/1388152.

Piedmont, R. (2004). Spiritual Transcendence as a Predictor of Psychosocial Outcome from an Outpatient Substance Abuse Program. *Psychology of Addictive Behaviors,* 18(3), 213-222.

Ramson, R.; Obert, J.; McCann, M.; & Ling, W. (2005). *Matrix Model.* Center City, MN: Hazelden.

Ridgway, P. (2009). *Nine passages on the journey of mental health recovery.* Handout Presented at Connecticut Department of Mental Health and Addiction Services Education and Training, Middletown, CT.

Ridgway, P.; McDiarmid, D.; Davidson, L.; Bayes, J.; Ratzloff, S. (2002). *Pathways to recovery.* University of Kansas: Supported Education Group, Kansas School of Welfare.

Rose, E.; Westefeld, J.; & Ansely, T. (2001). Spiritual issues in counseling: Clients' beliefs and preferences. *Journal of Counseling Psychology,* 48(1), 61-71.doi:10.1037/0022-0167.48.1.61.

Seeman, T.; Dubin, L.; & Seeman, M. (2003). Religiosity/ spirituality and health: A critical review of the evidence for biological pathways. *American Psychologist*, 58(1), 53-63. doi:10.1037/0003-066X.58.1.53.

Springborn, W. (1992). Steps 1-12. Minnesota City, MN: Hazelden.

Sullivan, W.P. (1998). Recoiling, regrouping, and recovering: First-person accounts of the role of spirituality in the course of serious mental illness. *New Directions of Mental Health Services.* Los Angeles: Josey-Bass Publishers.

Temple University; Spirituality protects against depression better than church attendance. (2008, November). *Psychology & Psychiatry Journal,* 9. Retrieved April 18, 2009, from ProQuest Psychology Journals database. (Document ID: 1590031151).

Twelve steps and twelve traditions. (2002). NY. World Service office.

UNIT 8/Ethics

Introduction

Our dual diagnosis dialogue would not be complete without a discourse in ethics as they relate to the field. Confidentiality/privacy shall be highlighted followed by an in-depth discussion of boundaries – crossings and violations – helpful and harmful! This area of discussion is not without varying opinions, philosophies, and controversy. The entry level counselor can get themselves into a difficult spot and at times, our decisions come back to haunt us. This unit is an attempt to provide safeguards and issues that will require some thought and principle.

CHAPTER 28

Confidentiality/Privacy

Confidentiality is an ethical obligation, whereas the privacy of privileged communication is a legal right and prevents clients' communication disclosed in court without their permission. State laws vary regarding privileged communication and counselors must learn the laws in their state.

Herlihy and Corey (1996) tell us that confidentiality is one of our most basic obligations. It is the foundation for clients' trust and ability to share with us openly. They need to know that the counselor is going to respect their innermost thoughts and secrets. Confidentiality is also one of the most problematic obligations we have. There are complex legal concerns, issues with new technology, communication complications with health care insurance companies, and our culture which places a high premium on privacy.

The American Counseling Association (ACA) devotes an entire section in its code of ethics to the subject of confidentiality (Section B). In sum, the counselor must "respect their clients' right to privacy and avoid illegal and unwarranted disclosures of confidential information" (B.1.a.).

Confidentiality needs to be discussed with the client at the beginning of treatment and as needed (B.1.g.), and to inform them what they reveal will be kept confidential except in certain circumstances:

1) It is sometimes permissible to discuss information with other counselors and experts, and in supervision in the interest of providing services to the client.
2) It is sometimes permissible to share information to protect someone who is in danger; i.e., child abuse or neglect, diminished capacity, or the elderly.
3) When there is imminent risk to client or others.
4) There is a legal duty to warn and protect a potential victim when a client threatens violence toward a person or persons.
5) In some cases, confidentiality cannot be guaranteed; in group therapy, in sessions with other people (family); if a client is a minor, if there is a court order.

Confidentiality also refers to the fact that the person is in treatment – period. A most common breach of confidentiality is when professionals are discussing cases amongst themselves when it may not really be pertinent to the client's interest; you know, for conversation sake. Also, we must be aware who is around us when we are discussing clients; can other people overhear us? Not only are communications confidential but so are records. Section B.4 of the American Counseling Association (ACA) Code of Ethics is about maintaining, storing, transferring, sharing, and disposing of records.

Comment for the Reader: Even with all the precautions, there are times when confidentiality gets broken. Examples are: 1) Two counselors get overheard talking in the hall about a client. 2) Someone in your group is friends with another group member's friend and says things they shouldn't 3) Something a client says at an AA meeting gets repeated. It is a horrible experience for the client, leaving them feeling violated. It's a betrayal of trust and can be difficult to undo the damage. Think. Why are you sharing this information about this client? Is it clinically related and in the interest of the client? Or is it out of curiosity, shoptalk, or even being sanctimonious? Where is the conversation taking place? Also, clients need lots of reminders and it makes for good trust-building to discuss it in groups frequently. We all need to know that our privacy is respected.

CHAPTER 29

Counselor/Client Relationships: Healthy Boundary Crossing and Harmful Boundary Violations

A discussion of boundaries and dual-relationships, that is, any other type of relationship with the client outside of the office, is vital. This is particularly true in rural areas where the counselor may be likely to run into the client often (he's the clerk at the supermarket) or have multiple roles with the client (her daughter is your daughter's best friend).

Also, the beginning counselor may be unaware of professional traps and getting in a jam that can come back to haunt them. They may not see the harm in extending the client/counselor relationship outside of the office. Some straight talk here. The role of the counselor can be a seductive one for counselor and client alike. The client is vulnerable and the counselor is powerful and seems to have all the answers. It can take training and experience to avoid some of the pitfalls of the profession. What follows is a frank discussion of what boundaries are and why they are important.

History and Trends. The earliest recognition that sexual relationships could be harmful to the client found its way into the Hippocratic Oath in the 5th century BC (Pope, 2001). The oath prohibits sex with patients. The code of the Nigerian Healing Arts, which was created before the Hippocratic Oath, did as well. Freud, considered to be the father of psychoanalysis/psychotherapy, also forbade it. In 1976, Roy vs. Hartogs, the first lawsuit brought against a therapist for sexual intercourse, based its theory of the harmful effects of sexual relations between a client and a therapist on Freud's writings. The taboo has continued into the 21st century and is probably more prevalent today than ever before.

The historic view on boundaries developed from transference theories with the perspective that the psychotherapy relationship is a transference-based relationship and with it an unbalanced power distribution (Barnett, 2007). Freud distinguished between the phenomenon of transference and what is otherwise considered as "falling in love" (Smith & Fitzpatrick, 1995). The client's feelings are a result of the analytic process not the personal charms of the therapist (Smith & Fitzpatrick, 1995). Psychotherapy is distinguished from other nonclinical activities. Legal history has determined that having sexual relationships with a client is abusing the role of transference and an abuse of trust in the therapeutic relationship. It is unacceptable behavior for the therapist, and this is held true for former clients, as well. Recently, the ACA code of ethics changed its principle from a 2-year restriction on relationships with former clients to 5 years (ACA code of ethics, 2005).

People come to the therapist in a vulnerable state of one sort or another. Whether it be from a mental illness; crisis; conflict; substance abuse; or family, medical, or legal issue, the client enjoys a special relationship with the therapist. A deep trust can develop as clients share things that might not otherwise be shared with anybody. The counselor may be viewed as many things: advisor, director, teacher, healer, consoler, comforter, and so forth. There is an inherent power in this role (Barnett, 2007). Pope (2001) cites research by Masters and Johnson that compared sex with a therapist as likened to rape, abuse, and incest. It exemplifies the broken trust and emotional dependence. Their study completed in the late 60s and early 70s reported surprising samples of clients who had sex with their therapists. Their studies were striking enough that Masters and Johnson supported charges of rape rather than malpractice, and believed that it should be built into the legal system as criminal and not civil.

Today, in many states, sex between a therapist and a client is illegal. Connecticut, for example, considers it to be sexual misconduct and assault. Sexual contact is distinguished from sexual intercourse. Consequences for sexual intercourse with a client are up to 10 years imprisonment, up to a $10,000 fine, and the loss of a public health license. Sexual contact may indicate license sanctions, or loss of license, up to 1-year imprisonment, and up to a $2,000 fine. The statutes also define a psychotherapist as a physician, psychologist, nurse, substance abuse counselor, social worker, marital and family therapist, and mental health service provider or anybody else, with or without a license that does psychotherapy. Psychotherapy is considered to be any kind of professional treatment, assessment, or counseling of any kind of mental or emotional condition (Connecticut statutes of sexual misconduct, n.d.).

Barnett (2007) suggests that therapists who are involved in sexual relationships with clients or former clients evolved into these relationships from lesser indiscretions. He indicates that dual relationships started with increasingly inappropriate behaviors that the therapist thought harmless when viewed in isolation.

Interestingly enough, Pope (n.d.) cites Gutheil who discusses Freud as setting the standard for boundaries. He reports how Freud himself sent letters to his clients, lent them books, gave gifts, shared news about his family, shared meals, took walks with clients, and analyzed his own daughter.

This resembles some habits of humanistic counselors who engage in what some consider gross neglect of client-therapist boundaries, such as self-disclosure and hugging at the end of a session (Williams, 1997). Williams (1997) cites Bugental's (1987) humanistic perspective suggesting that a client and therapist may be said to have a true bonding relationship after long-term treatment of sharing "warm communion and great stress." He calls this a love relationship and states it is nothing less. Furthermore, that client and therapist are partners and endure great difficulty and reward, and that it is "unreal to expect otherwise" (Williams, 1997).

Boundaries. Boundaries are the rules of the game between the therapist and the client (Knapp & Slattery, 2004). They distinguish the therapeutic relationship, or professional, business relationship from a social relationship. The rules clarify and define what is acceptable in therapy as opposed to other types of relationships. These rules are also referred to as the 'therapeutic frame' to describe the structure of the therapy relationship and provide borders to keep within. There is general agreement that boundaries help to create a safe and reliable atmosphere for the client to take part in mental and emotional work. However, there is also controversy as to what is appropriate and in-bounds or inappropriate or out-of-bounds in the context of therapy (Johnston & Farber, 1996).

What exactly are the issues? They include, but are not limited to: hugging, eating out with, self-disclosing, making house calls, visiting in the hospital, exchanging gifts, engaging in non-sexual socializing with, lending books, extending sessions, and making financial concessions (Williams, 1997). Some rules regarding boundaries are absolute (Knapp & Slattery, 2004). The Code of Ethics, of both the APA and the ACA and no doubt numerous other governing bodies, prohibits sexual relationships with current clients. This extends to those family members and others close to the client, and there are specifications regarding former clients. The ACA formerly put a 2-year restriction on relationships with clients and recently changed it to 5 years. The APA permits it under highly unusual circumstances. Some standards are more flexible depending on the context and duration of the relationship, for example.

The sexual boundary issue revolves around what is considered 'transference abuse' (Williams, 1997). Transference is a phenomenon in psychology characterized by an unconscious redirection of feelings for one person to another. In a therapy context, transference refers to redirection of a client's feelings from a significant person to a therapist. Transference was first described by Sigmund Freud, who acknowledged its importance for psychoanalysis to better understand the patient's feelings. Often the client places the therapist in a god-like or guru status (Corey, 1986). From a Freudian perspective, a therapist's attraction to a client was first seen as a reaction to the client's transference (Pope, Tabachnik, & Keith-Speige, n.d.). Sexual misconduct laws use transference as the basis of the violation. Imbedded in trust issues between client and therapist is the nature of power in the relationship.

There is an inherent imbalance of power in the therapy relationship, particularly those therapists that rely on psychoanalysis as a basis (Barrett, 2007). The therapist is in a much more powerful and influential position than the client who comes into therapy looking for help and trusting and dependent on the therapist. The client trusts that the therapist, a trained professional, is directing his/her skills toward the needs of the client. The relationship by nature is one sided with the focus being on the client, his needs, fears, thoughts, feelings, and experiences. They may share information that is not shared with parent, spouse, significant other, friend, clergy, or anyone. And they do this with the goal of receiving help and the relief of emotional pain and crisis. For the therapist to use this trust and power for personal gain, or to meet personal needs, is a violation. Whether this is intentional or not, the therapist is completely responsible for what occurs (Barrett, 2007). This is a fundamental professional standard. In order to avoid harm, a number of boundaries are recognized to establish the professional relationship.

Williams (1997) recommends a rationale for careful boundaries. He purports that first, psychotherapy is a powerful vehicle that generates powerful emotions. Victims of sexual client-therapist relationships are mostly women. Male therapists have a much higher rate of violating boundaries. Psychotherapy clients often revert to very vulnerable states. This regression is similar to that of a parent-child relationship. As a result, the male therapist, the 'father' must ensure that the vulnerability of the female client is safeguarded. The message must be clear that this vulnerability will not be violated. This message comes in the form of boundaries, such as scheduling or billing issues, touching, self-disclosing, and social contact. It is essential to reminding the client that this is a professional relationship and not an intimate, sexual, or social relationship. Clients, because of their vulnerable state, may experience emotions that feel more intimate, sexual, or social, and may initiate such behavior. It is solely the responsibility of the therapist to maintain the professional relationship by setting limits. Some clients, because of transference issues and previous experiences may interpret harmless mention of a social or personal nature as intimate, sexual, or social. These are to be avoided in order to prevent any confusion as to the nature of the relationship. Due to this context for the client, seemingly harmless boundary-crossing can be a sign of negligence because of the bigger misguided message it sends to the client.

Gottlieb (n.d.) cites Gonsiorek and Brown (1989) who make a distinction between two types of therapy. One is when the transferential relationship plays a significant role. On the other hand, sometimes therapy is short term and there is insufficient time for transference to develop.

I will deal more with sexual relationships further in this chapter. There are less clear- cut situations, however, that come up in the client-therapist relationship, and not all therapists use transference as the basis for therapy . . . many do not subscribe to the concept.

The opposing perspective contends that rigorous boundaries are excessive and are ineffective for a large number of clients. The argument is that it depends on the psychological experience for both the client and the therapist. What may appear to be a boundary violation in one context might be experienced as strong and comforting to another client. One therapist might be concerned with maintaining emotional distance in the professional relationship, while another is strong and compassionate in a client's despairing moments. Johnston and Farber (1996) discuss clients who cite situations where the therapist stepped out of role as the most memorable and significant. They suggest the controversy over boundaries should be about what makes therapy successful.

Humanistic, behavioral and other eclectic psychotherapies are influenced by other concepts and methods other than Freud's psychoanalytic concept of transference that might be construed as gross violations of boundaries. Humanistic psychotherapy is directed at breaking down boundaries between client and therapist, or not maintaining them (Corey, 1986; Williams, 1997). Person-centered therapy is about the authentic encounter between the client and the therapist. The basic premise is that significant positive change can only occur in the context of a congruent, genuine relationship that contains unconditional positive regard and acceptance for the client, and accurate empathic understanding (Corey, 1986). Rogers hypothesized that no other conditions are necessary. Client change is based on this type of therapeutic relationship or alliance, and the ground rules may be different and more flexible than what has previously been described.

Williams (1997) quotes Bugental (1987) who purports that long-term treatment that has contained a good degree of depth, inevitably includes moments of 'warm communion' as well as periods of great stress for both client and therapist. Furthermore, there is a true bonding which takes place (which is not always recognized by those who subscribe to more objective practices), and the client and therapist can experience a type of love relationship which is not by any means simply explained as transference and counter-transference. The client and therapist are partners in a difficult, sometimes perilous yet rewarding, experience.

Humanistic therapists openly share their thoughts and feelings responsibly and authentically, discuss reasons why they do things, and acknowledge difficulties. It is believed this can be accomplished without harm to the client, in fact will help him. Humanists maintain that much psychoanalytic doctrine contains unnecessary prohibitions. If the client is encouraged to call the therapist by his first name, socializing might occur – especially in a treatment center. A therapist might attend a wedding or visit a client in the hospital. Gift-giving is not unheard of and hugging is not unusual. Humanist theories do not specifically endorse any of these; however, they are done openly and innocuously and flourish in a spontaneous atmosphere. For a genuine experience to occur between client and therapist, and thus authentic growth for the client, there must be a shared experience (Williams, 1997).

Williams (1997) quotes Lazarus, a behavior therapist, as indicating psychoanalysis as 'speculative' and transference as a 'myth.' The psychoanalyst does not disclose because he wishes to be a blank screen for the client to project his own ideas onto. The behaviorist, to the contrary, shares his views, thoughts, and feelings in order for 'modeling' to occur where the client can copy the therapist's behavior or attitudes. This can be curative.

Dual Relationships and Decision-Making. Younggren (n.d.) outlines some of the thinking that should go into the consideration of a dual relationship. Generally speaking, it is not the existence alone of a dual relationship that is problematic. Difficulty and controversy arise as a result of outcomes. This discussion will reflect the welfare of the client, but will also review safeguards for the professional. As a rule, it is likely in the therapists' interest to avoid any dual relationships if possible. It is well known that in some rural areas, dual relationships are completely unavoidable (Slattery, 2005).

There are questions the therapist must ask himself before engaging in a dual relationship to ensure it is in the best interest of both the client and the relationship. First, is this relationship necessary? Therapy is difficult enough without bringing other factors into it. Next, is the relationship exploitive? If this is not clear, then the therapist must ask himself, who does the relationship benefit? Or, perhaps more clearly, is there a risk there could be harm to the client? Will the therapeutic relationship be damaged as a result of the dual relationship? These questions my not be easily answered, but the therapist has an obligation to be in touch with risk factors. Furthermore, they must be asked continually throughout treatment. Lastly, the therapist must ask himself if he is being objective in the evaluation of this matter. This may require consulting with other individuals; perhaps peers, and/or an attorney. It is good practice to adequately document the decision process in treatment records.

At this venture, this paper distinguishes between boundary 'crossing' – neutral or helpful vs. boundary 'violations' – harmful (Pope, n.d.). Pope (n.d.) and Sonne (n.d.) discuss basic assumptions regarding ethical awareness used in decision-making. The therapist needs continual awareness of the ethical implications of his actions. This is an ongoing process. Therapists can get overwhelmed, dulled, distracted, and drained, and perceptions are affected accordingly. Codes of Ethics guide us, but are not a substitute for thinking things through. Every client is different. Every therapist is different. Every situation is different. Ethical dilemmas occur all the time. The research is evolving and the therapist has a responsibility to stay abreast of it. The overwhelming majority of therapists keep high ethical standards, but everyone is fallible and it is important to remember this. The most seasoned therapist may hold close to a belief that is misguided. The therapist must always be asking himself if he is missing something. It is a red flag if the therapist spends more time looking at the practices of others rather than his own. Pope encourages the therapist not to just look into things he is unaware of, but to look at the things he is sure of, and to remember there are often on-the-spot decisions. There is no valid way to avoid ethical struggles. Lastly, consultation is highly encouraged to weigh out decisions and their consequences (Pope & Keith-Speigal, n.d.).

When making decisions involving boundaries, the therapist must ask himself 'what is the best possible outcome and the worst possible outcome' (Pope, n.d.). If there is potential harm, are there ways to address it? Consider the research as a driving force of the direction of things. Pope (n.d.) encourages having at least one associate that one can discuss boundary issues with. He encourages paying attention to uncomfortable feelings, and understand what they may be about. It is important to refer a client to another peer if the therapist, for whatever reason, feels he cannot work with the client effectively.

Pope (n.d.) has observed several cognitive errors that occur in the decisions that lead to boundary violations. It is a mistaken notion, for example, that what happens outside of the office has nothing to do with therapy. Consider the example of the client who is also a student, and looks for favors on a paper deadline due to her anxiety. Another fallacy is thinking that crossing a boundary with a client is the same as doing the same thing with someone who is not a client. For example, the gesture of helping a client on with her coat, lending a client a sweater because it is cold in the office, offering a ride because it is raining, could be taken differently by cients. Everyday acts may have unintended effects as an act of friendship or a romantic gesture. Age and gender can affect interpretations, as well. For example, the young female client who is told by the therapist she looks lovely today – may have different meanings if the therapist is male or female.

Another error in thinking is the therapist believing that his understanding of a boundary crossing is the same as the client's understanding. For example, the therapist may put his arm around the client who just lost her father, thinking it to be a helpful and consoling gesture – and the client goes stiff. Along the same vein, the therapist may believe that a boundary crossing that was beneficial for one client will be beneficial for another. For example, bartering may work with one client but produce an indignant response from another.

Often the therapist may believe a boundary crossing is an isolated situation. For example, the therapist brings in left-over brownies from home to use them up, and offers one to a client. The next week the client comes in with coffee and pastry for the two of them to share.

Another fallacy is that if the therapist is feeling certain that there is no conflict of interest, no consequences, no risks or downside – then there aren't any. It is easy to deceive ourselves or simply not have thought of all the circumstances.

Some therapists believe that self-disclosure is always useful because it shows congruency and trust. Self-disclosure may not always be wanted by the client or simply may not always be appropriate.

Sexual Issues. It has been discussed in the history section of this paper about the vulnerable state that clients come into therapy with, and much space has been devoted to describing the sacred trust that develops between client and therapist. The discussion from a humanist perspective emphasized the value of the therapeutic alliance in treatment for the client to make changes. The differences between what are boundary crossings and boundary violations are herein. This last section concerns the most common reactions that are frequently associated with client-therapist sex.

One common reaction is one of extreme ambivalence and may be very debilitating. The client can be caught between two compelling impulses: one to escape from the relationship, and the other to continue to foster it and cling to the therapist. Some clients experience cognitive dysfunction whether the sex began before or after the termination of therapy. This can be experienced as difficulty with attention, memory, and concentration. Some clients' have unwanted thoughts, intrusive images, flashbacks, or nightmares. They may interfere with client's ability to work, be social, or carry out routine. Similar to cognitive dysfunction is emotional lability. This can be severe and disruptive emotions that may come out seemingly without cause. The client may feel helpless and out of control (Pope, n.d.).

The client may experience a sense of emptiness, as if a part of them is lost. This can be accompanied by a sense of isolation and can feel overwhelming and horrifying. Often clients have an irrational sense of guilt. It is irrational because it is the therapists' responsibility to avoid sexual relations with the client which is considered sexual abuse, and clients' experiences are likened to incest, abuse, and rape victims (Pope, n.d.).

The client may emerge from the relationship with an impaired ability to trust. Therapy rests on a foundation of trust. Clients come into a stranger's office and begin talking about thoughts, feelings, fears, and impulses that they would not discuss with anyone else. Every state appreciates the sensitive and sacred nature of these disclosures and have established laws regarding client-therapist privilege. Aside from trusting the therapist to protect their innermost soul, the client trusts the therapist to act in a way that will keep them safe from harm personally, ethically, and legally. The trust has been violated (Pope, n.d.).

Some clients experience an increased risk for suicide. Research suggests that 14% of these clients attempt suicide, and that one in a hundred clients involved sexually with a therapist commit suicide (Pope, n.d.).

Clients may experience boundary confusion. In legitimate therapy, the therapeutic alliance and process continues in the office, between sessions and after termination. Violating these boundaries can have long-term effects on the roles and boundaries that people use in other areas (Pope, n.d.).

Many clients suffer from sexual confusion following a sexual relationship with a therapist. Clients have reported feeling disgusted with their sexual impulses and behavior, and have expressed cautiousness about their sexual feelings. Especially when coupled with feelings of guilt, emptiness, and isolation, some clients engage in other sexual relationships that support their guilty worthless feelings (Pope, n.d.).

Many clients who have been in a sexual relationship with a therapist have justifiable anger, but they may experience difficulty expressing it. Some clients report feeling numb. Some report feeling anger at themselves (Pope, n.d.).

On a different slant, but interestingly enough, in a study by Pope, Leveson, and Schover (n.d.), 2% of respondents answered affirmatively to the statement, " I believe that sexual relationships between students and their psychology teachers, administrators, or clinical supervisors, can be beneficial to both parties."

Assumptions. Early biomedical ethics assert the principles of non-maleficence and beneficence; doing no harm and promoting good for the welfare of the client (Beauchamp & Childress, 2001). Early Freudian psychoanalysis promulgated theories of transference and counter-transference. The Humanistic and Behavioral perspective of therapy created a different style of therapy that is more interactive. While these have been influential forces in psychology, they have not overshadowed the Freudian foundations of psychoanalysis. The literature indicates that in the 1960s and 1970s there was a swing toward more liberal-minded boundaries with clients. However, the pendulum has swung back in the 1990s and 2000s into a period of enhanced accountability of the part of therapists.

Concurrently, there has been a paradigm shift to client-centered therapy in which the client has an integral role in their treatment planning, tasks, and goals. The therapist's role is more one of partner and collaborator than 'expert.' Nonetheless, this does not seem to have modified the professional boundaries as set forth in Codes of Ethics; at least not in the way humanistic and behavioral theories, methods, and techniques did.

However, there seems to be a tolerance for looser boundaries in some therapy settings: gift-giving, hugging, lending items, possible out of office visits (hospital or home), dual relationships, and other seeming transgressions of boundaries. There is a school of thought that these boundary crossings may be beneficial to the client. The proof is left to the outcome and the burden is on the therapist to have documented supportive decision-making. Otherwise, the trend is conservative and lends toward caution and the client's interest, safety, and well-being is paramount.

In summation, the lines have been drawn; traditionalists supporting firm and formal boundaries on the one side and humanistic/behaviorist supporters on the other. There is room for more than one theory, but this is an age of accountability. The question will rest on what is in the best interest of the client? And the test is what makes for successful outcomes? These questions will create future research, and theory will follow. For example, if hugging is beneficial in certain cases or situations with certain clients, research might look at when is this so, and what type of client is likely to benefit. Under what conditions is a hug likely to be detrimental? The big picture includes precautions the therapist must take to avoid misinterpretation, misunderstanding, and any potential harm to the client while maximizing potential good for the welfare of the client.

The Recovering Counselor

When counselors themselves are in recovery, it can pose unique problems when living in the same community as their clients. In particular, if and when the counselor and client attend the same 12-step meeting, there are special considerations.

First, it is necessary for counselors to have their own recovery program, and it can be a conflict of interest if the counselor was to share certain personal information at the same meeting with the client. It can, in some instances, compromise the counselor/client relationship by affecting the dynamics involved. The client may no longer view the counselor in a professional regard, because boundaries have been crossed; this can affect the efficacy of the client's treatment. The best-case scenario is for the counselor to keep his program separate and distinct from the client.

It is also possible that a well-integrated counselor, sharing at a meeting, only serves to enhance their role as a model for the client. In essence, the individual seen at the meeting is an extension of the counselor seen in the office. A problem arises if the counselor's privacy is inhibited or the nature of this dual relationship adversely affects the client in any way.

In most cases, such a conflict can be avoided. However, in small communities or in rural areas, it may be more difficult. The potential awkwardness or conflict of interest should not be ignored, but discussed with a supervisor or peer, and in some cases, the client wants to find a workable resolution which would depend on the individual situation.

Conclusion

Ethics are a topic that many take for granted, but it is easy to find oneself in a dilemma and it is to be expected. Situations arise all the time. The important thing is that when we have that first sense that something does not feel quite right, we must pay attention to it. Often the best thing may be to discuss it with a peer or supervisor to determine the appropriate response, if any. These things come up all the time: confidentiality may get treated somewhat casually, dual-relationships may occur, the counselor may find they have strong feelings regarding a client, and so forth. The issue is usually how we deal with it before anything becomes a problem. Our decisions and conduct reflect on ourselves, our agency, and have ramifications for our clients. Nonetheless, the best advice I can provide the early counselor with, is that you have to protect yourself. Listen to yourself. You will know if something is not quite right or you are uncertain about. We do have to be careful and look at things as they arise before a situation, whatever it is, may get out of hand.

UNIT 8 Highlights

CH 28: Confidentiality/Privacy

- Confidentiality/ethical obligation
- Privacy/legal right based on privileged communication
- Exceptions/medical emergency/child or elder abuse/ imminent risk to self or others, including duty to warn/ court order

CH 29: Boundaries

- Healthy boundary crossing/harmful boundary violation
- History/origin Hippocratic Oath 500 BC
- Boundary Violations/sexual relations/transference violation/ client vulnerable/counselor powerful/criminal
- Boundary crossings/acceptable vs. unacceptable/ self-disclosure/hugging/hospital visit/attending wedding
- Humanistic/behavioral and other eclectic therapies do not subscribe to transference/serve to break down client-counselor barriers
- Key questions/who is benefitting?/Is it exploitive?
- Recovering Counselor/needs own program/potential conflict of interest/seek supervision

Study Guide

1) Why is confidentiality essential to the counseling process?
2) What are exceptions to maintaining confidentiality?
3) Describe your boundaries with your clients. Do you lean toward a conventional conservative approach? Or do you lean toward more liberal humanistic perspectives?
4) Would you . . . hug a client? Have lunch with a client? Attend a client's wedding? Visit a client in the hospital? Have a relationship with a former client? If you are in recovery, would you attend a meeting that a client was also attending? Why? Why not?

References

ACA Code of Ethics as approved by the ACA governing council. (2005). Retrieved from http://www.counseling.org on April 15, 2008.

Barnett, J. (2007). Whose boundaries are they anyway? *Professional Psychology: Research and Practice,* 38(4), 401-405.

Beauchamp, T.L. & Childress, J.F. (2006). *Principles of biomedical ethics* (5th ed.). New York: Oxford University Press.

Corey, G. (1986). *Theory and practice of counseling and psychotherapy* (3rd ed.). Belmont, CA: Wadsworth, Inc.

Corey, G. & Herlihy, B. (1996). *ACA Ethical standards casebook* (5th ed.). Alexandria, VA: American Counseling Association.

Connecticut State Statute on Sexual Misconduct for psychotherapists. (n.d.). Retrieved from http://www.cassw.org/documents/Connecticut%20State%20Statute%20on%20Sexual%20Misconduct.pdf – on April 15, 2008.

Glickauf-Hughes, C. & Chance, S. ((1995). Answering clients' questions. *Psychotherapy: Theory, Research, Practice, Training,* (32), 3, 375-380.

Gottlieb, M. C. (n.d.). Dual relationships avoiding exploitive dual relationships: A decision-making model. Retrieved from http://kspope.com/dual/gottlieb.php on April 15, 2008.

Hamilton, J. & Spruill, J. (1999). Identifying and reducing risk factors related to trainee-client sexual misconduct. *Professional Psychology: Research and Practice,* (30), 3, 318-327.

Johnston, S. & Farber, B. (1996). The maintenance of boundaries in psychotherapeutic practice. *Psychotherapy: Theory, Research, Practice, Training,* (33), 3, 391-402.

Knapp, S. & Slattery, J. (2004). Professional boundaries in non-traditional settings. Professional Psychology: Research and Practice, (35), 5, 553-558.

Lamb, D.H.; Catanzaro, S.J.; & Moorman, A.S. (2004). A preliminary look at how psychologists identify, evaluate, and proceed with possible multiple relationship dilemmas. *Professional Psychology: Research and Practice,* (35), 3, 248-254.

Luchner, A.F.; Miralimi, H.; Moser, C.J.; & Jones, R.A. (2008). Maintaining boundaries in psychotherapy: covert narcissistic personality characteristics and psychotherapists. *Psychotherapy: Theory, Research, Practice, Training,* (45), 1, 1-14.

Pope, K.S. (n.d.). *How the field began to focus on distinguishing boundary crossings (helpful or neutral) from boundary violations (harmful) in the early 1990s.* Retrieved from http://kspope.com/dual/Gutheil.php on April 15, 2008.

Pope, K.S. (n.d.). *Sex between therapists and clients.* Retrieved from http://kspope.com/sexiss/sexencyc.php on April 20, 2008.

Pope, K.S. & Keith-Speigal, P. (n.d.). *A practical approach to boundaries in psychotherapy: Making decisions, bypassing blunders, and mending fences.* Retrieved from http://kspope.com/ethics/boundaries.php on April 15, 2008.

Pope, K.S.; Levenson, H.; & Schover L.R. (n.d.) *Sexual intimacy in psychology training: Results and implications of a national survey.* Retrieved from http://kspope.com/sexiss/research1.php on April 15, 2008.

Pope, K.S. (n.d.). 21 Ethical fallacies: cognitive strategies to justify unethical behavior. Retrieved from http://kspope.com/ethics/ethicalstandards.php on April 15, 2008.

Pope, K.S.; Tabachnik, B.G.; & Keith-Spiege, P. (n.d.). *Sexual attraction to clients: The human therapist and the (sometimes) inhuman training system.* Retrieved from http://kspope.com/sexiss/research5.php on April 15, 2008.

Slattery, J. (2005). Preventing role slippage during work in the community: Guidelines for new psychologists and supervisees. *Psychotherapy: Theory, Research, Practice, Training,* (42), 3, 384-394.

Smith, D. & Fitzpatrick, M. (1995). Patient-therapist boundary issues: An integrative review of theory and research. *Professional Psychology: Research and Practice,* 26(5), 499-506.

Williams, M. (1997). Boundary violations: Do some contended standards of care fail to encompass commonplace procedures of humanistic, behavioral, and eclectic psychotherapies? *Psychotherapy: Theory, Research, Practice, Training,* 34(3), 238-249.

UNIT 9/CONCLUSION

CHAPTER 30

Closing Comment for the Reader

IT IS MY HOPE THAT YOUR ACADEMIC ACCOMPLISHMENTS add to your personal and professional pursuits, and that in some small way, this dialogue has contributed. To that end, let me summarize what I hope you will take away from it.

I strongly believe, that the most important thing we, as counselors, can provide the client with is a working alliance. We need to provide them with a climate to grow in. . . and the answers will come. The therapeutic alliance/relationship can help the client assume responsibility for their recovery. Believe in the client's ability to uncover what works for them and to find their own answers – (but, we can help!).

It is important to understand the Strengths-Based Paradigm, which supports the client wherever they are in relation to recovery, and respects them in the collaborative process of treatment. This is how harm-reduction theory can be useful.

Medications are a tool for the toolbox. Many clients require a medication awakening before they can experience a spiritual awakening.

Find a counseling approach that you are comfortable with and that fits your perspective and style. Then work on developing a more eclectic approach by being able to draw on various methods from various other theories. Different approaches are going to be useful as different things are going to work for different clients, and we want to be versatile.

It makes sense to address dual diagnoses as integrated treatment because the client comes to us with an integrated substance abuse and mental health issue. It is a disservice to the client to attempt to separate them out. It's my belief that all substance abusers are dual diagnosed; it is just a matter of relative degree. A client may come in with a 'soft' anxiety disorder or depressive disorder, but they are most likely self-medicating nonetheless. In other words, they are no doubt getting many needs met by drugging, and usually it becomes the main, if not the only, coping mechanism.

While 12-Step programs are not the only answer – and that was certainly repeated enough times throughout – there are two (probably more) components from AA that are vital to recovery, whatever form that make take. 1) Recovery has to involve changes; changes in thought, feeling, and behavior. 2) There needs to be a spiritual component. Don't let your clients throw you off by the word "spiritual;" we can call it many things. Anything that enhances positive growth and way of life is going to have a spiritual nature to it.

It is also my hope that an understanding of the Stages of Spirituality will assist you in helping the client to develop that positive growth and positive way of life. It is true that the dual-diagnosed individuals who participated attend 12-Step programs. I am a fan. Can you tell?

Glossary

Dual diagnosis – a substance use disorder, plus another mental health disorder that impact upon each other.

Co-occurring disorders – see dual diagnosis.

Substance abuse – a maladaptive pattern of substance use leading to significant impairment or distress.

Substance dependence – the distinction between abuse and dependence is one of compulsion; dependence includes withdrawal and tolerance.

Addiction – see substance dependence.

Disease model – or medical model; chronic, progressive, incurable, uncontrollable AOD usage; a result of genetic, brain, and anatomic chemistry.

Medical model – ses disease model.

Alcoholics Anonymous – a recovery program based on a process of change, utilizing a 12-step model leading toward psychic change and spiritual awakening.

Harm reduction theory – AOD treatment approach including theories of reduced drug usage, reduced frequency of drug usage, and reduced harm based on usage.

Psychodynamic theory – based on personality development, Freud philosophy; includes focus on unconscious processes.

Cognitive behaviorism – therapy that stresses the role of thinking and beliefs on behavior.

Behavior therapy – based on learning principles and resolution to maladaptive behavior patterns.

Humanistic/Phenomenological Theory – focuses on the self and one's experiences based on freedom to choose one's behavior, and client's capacity to solve their own issues and self-actualize.

Existential therapy – therapy based on attempting to find meaning in what might be a meaningless world (Frankl, May, Yalom).

Gestalt Therapy – experiential therapy based on awareness and integration (Perls).

Reality Therapy – treatment based on freedom of choice and self-responsibility; client learns to meet their own needs (Glasser).

Narrative Therapy – a treatment approach based upon one's story, and how one's perception impacts one's life (Payne).

Person-centered Therapy – therapy based on the therapeutic alliance and client's ability to solve their issues, given the right environment (Rogers).

Attending – in individual counseling; simply paying attention to the client and being observant; eye contact.

Paraphrasing – in individual counseling; restating the client's message in different words.

Reflection – in individual counseling; paraphrasing and including emotional tone in client's message.

Clarification – in individual counseling; seeking clarity to client's confusing message.

Leading – in individual counseling; directly or indirectly encouraging the client to continue elaborating.

Summarization – in individual counseling; integration of client's feelings and ideas, and repeated back to client.

Support – in individual counseling; letting the client know you understand what they are saying and that their feelings are not uncommon.

Approval – in individual counseling; expressing agreement with client's thoughts, feelings, or actions.

Confrontation – therapist's honest reaction to client's thoughts, feelings, or actions that appear in conflict or in discrepancy.

Interpretation – presenting the client with counselor's understanding of the meaning of client's thoughts, feeling, actions.

Information – in the role of educator or consultant, providing pertinent data to client.

Instruction – teaching the client new coping skills or other appropriate behavior.

Stages of change – the process of change, including 1) precontemplative stage = not ready to make changes 2) contemplative stage = beginning to think about making changes 3) preparation stage = considering change, but unsure yet how to go about it 4) action stage = actively putting changes into motion 5) maintenance = continuing to implement positive behaviors that are working.

Precontemplation stage – see stages of change.

Contemplation stage– see stages of change.

Preparation stage– see stages of change.

Action stage– see stages of change.

Maintenance stage– see stages of change.

Motivational interviewing – inspiring recovery by utilizing and supporting client strengths and goals, collaborating with client objectives, and the use of motivating interview skills.

Neurosis – classification of mental functioning involving distressful and dysfunctional behavior.

Psychosis – classification of mental functioning involving distressful and dysfunctional behavior including delusions and/or verbal and/or visual.

Generalized Anxiety disorder – at least 6 months of persistent and excessive anxiety and worry (APA, 2004).

Post traumatic stress disorder – re-experiencing of an extremely traumatic event accompanied by symptoms of increased arousal and by avoidance of stimuli associated with the trauma (APA, 2004).

Panic disorder – sudden onset of intense apprehension, fearfulness, or terror, often associated with feelings of impending doom; may be accompanied by such symptoms as shortness of breath, palpitations, chest pain or discomfort, and fear of "going crazy" or losing control (APA, 2004).

Agoraphobia – anxiety about or avoidance of, places or situations from which escape might be difficult or embarrassing, or in which help may not be available in the event of a panic attack (APA, 2004).

Obsessive compulsive disorder – characterized by obsessions which cause marked anxiety or distress and/or by compulsions which serve to neutralize anxiety (APA, 2004).

Major depression – two years of depressed mood for more days than not, and at least four additional symptoms of depression (APA, 2004).

Bipolar – characterized by one or more manic or mixed episodes usually accompanied by major depressive episodes (APA, 2004).

Dysthymia – characterized by two years of depressed mood for more days than not, accompanied by additional depressive symptoms that do not meet criteria for a major depressive disorder (APA, 2004).

Attention deficit disorder/Hyperactivity – characterized by prominent symptoms of inattention and/or hyperactive impulsivity (APA, 2004).

Schizophrenia – disorder that lasts at least six months and includes at least one month of active-phase (with two or more of: delusions, hallucinations, disorganized speech, grossly disorganized or catatonic behavior (APA, 2004).

Personality disorders – an enduring pattern of inner experience and behavior that deviates markedly from the expectations of the individual's culture; is pervasive and inflexible (APA, 2004).

Paradigm – underlying theories and methodology of a scientific model.

Neurotransmitters – microscopic bits of chemicals that contain messages to the nervous system. (Inaba & Cohen, 2000).

Serotonin – major neurotransmitter that helps control mood stability.

Noreprenephrine – major neurotransmitter that helps control motivation, hunger, attention span, confidence, and alertness.

Dopamine – major neurotransmitter that helps control motor activity, emotional stability, satiation, and the reward/reinforcement center.

12 Steps – the foundation of Alcoholics Anonymous and various other spin-offs which form a program of psychic change and potential spiritual awakening.

transference – a client-therapist relationship dynamic in which the client's unfinished business with a mother, father, or other significant person in their lives manifests itself in the relationship and distorts the present (Corey, 2009).

counter transference – the irrational reaction the therapist may have in relation to the client that may interfere with their objectivity (Corey, 2009).

DSM – diagnostic statistical manual; psychiatric reference book of classifications, categories, descriptions, and criteria of mental health diagnostics.

nos – not otherwise specified; categorical term used in the DSM when a diagnosis does not fit specific criteria of categorical diagnostics.

stimulants – uppers: central nervous system stimulants includes cocaine (crack, freebase), amphetamines (crystal, seed, crank, ice), Ritalin, adderall – creates energized muscle system, increased heart rate and blood pressure, insomnia, decreased appetite (Inaba & Cohen, 2000).

depressants – downers: central nervous system depressants include opiates (opium, morphine, codeine, heroin, methadone, oxycodone, vicodin; sedatives, hypnotics (benzodiazepines – xanax, valium/barbituates): alcohol (beer, wine, hard liquor); others (lookalikes, muscle relaxants, bromides) (Inaba & Cohen, 2000).

psychedelics – hallucinogens: substances that produce distorted perceptions and induce illusions (LSD, psilocybin, mushrooms, MDMA [ecstacy], MDA), belladonna, cannabinoids (marijuana, hashish): others (ketamine, PCP) (Inaba & Cohen, 2000).

inhalants – deliriants: gaseous or liquid substances that are inhaled and absorbed through the lungs including solvents, glue, gasoline, paints, STP, hosehold sprays, nitrates (amyl nitrate, butyl nitrate) nitrous oxide (laughing gas) (Inaba & Cohen, 2000).

sports drugs – anabolic steroids (performance-enhancing drugs), Human growth Hormone (HGH), herbal/nutritional supplements – creatine, amphetaline, pain killers, beta blockers (Inaba & Cohen, 2000).

central nervous system – half of the nervous sytem (brain, spinal cord).

peripheral nervous system – half of the nervous system (it connects the CNS with internal/external environments (Inaba & Cohen, 2000).

old brain – the primal brain; brain stem, cerebellum, limbic system (regulates physiological functions, brain emotions and cravings, imprints survival memories (Inaba & Cohen, 2000).

new brain – neocortex; (functions to speak, reason, create, and remember).

post acute withdrawal syndrome – a recurrence of the addiction withdrawal symptoms which can trigger cravings.

anti-psychotic medication – drugs used to treat psychosis which block dopamine (haldol, thorazine, mellaril, prolixin, risperidol, zyprexa, clozaril, abilify).

anti-depressants – drugs used to treat depression by correcting imbalance of serotonin, dopamine and noreprinephrine (prozac, paxil, zoloft, lexapro, celexa, wellbutrin, effexor).

INDEX

C

D

E

I

J

L

M

N

O

P

R

S

T

V

W

Y

Z

CPSIA information can be obtained at www.ICGtesting.com
Printed in the USA
236702LV00003B/27/P

9 781450 756785